READY-SET-REVIEW

F.A. Davis ... lphia

Kathleen A. Ohman
Professor of Nursi...
College of St. Bene...
St. John's University
St. Joseph, Minneso...

NCLEX-RN®
Alternate-Format

Q&A

F. A. Davis Company
1915 Arch Street
Philadelphia, PA 19103
www.fadavis.com

Printed in China

Last digit indicates print number: 10 9 8 7 6 5 4 3 2 1

Publisher, Nursing: Robert G. Martone
Director of Content Development: Darlene D. Pedersen
Sr. Project/NCLEX Editor: Padraic J. Maroney
Design and Illustration Manager: Carolyn O'Brien
Consultants: Elizabeth Cohn, RN, ACNP, DNSc; Aida L. Egues, RN, DNP, RN, APHN-BC, PHCNS-BC, CNE; Robin Gallagher, PhD, CRNP; Delores B. Lawson, DSN, RN; Maria A. Marconi, MS, RN; Jana McCallister, PhD(c), RN; Tracey S. Merworth, MSN, RN; Elizabeth J. Murray, PhD, RN, CNE; Lisa South, RN, DSN; Jo A. Voss, PhD, RN, CNS; Kelly N. White, MSN, FNP-BC; Ester Wilkinson, MSN, FNP; Joyce A. Wright, PhD, RN, CNL

As new scientific information becomes available through basic and clinical research, recommended treatments and drug therapies undergo changes. The author(s) and publisher have done everything possible to make this book accurate, up to date, and in accord with accepted standards at the time of publication. The author(s), editors, and publisher are not responsible for errors or omissions or for consequences from application of the book, and make no warranty, expressed or implied, in regard to the contents of the book. Any practice described in this book should be applied by the reader in accordance with professional standards of care used in regard to the unique circumstances that may apply in each situation. The reader is advised always to check product information (package inserts) for changes and new information regarding dose and contraindications before administering any drug. Caution is especially urged when using new or infrequently ordered drugs.

Table of Contents

Tab 1 Safe and Effective Care Environment | Management of Care

Test 1: Management of Care: Ethical, Legal, and Safety Issues in Nursing

1. A nurse is accessing a client's electronic medical record in the client's room to administer medications. Which steps should the nurse take to access the client's electronic medication administration record (eMar) to administer and document the medications? Place each step in the correct numerical order (1–7).

_____ 1. Determine if the medical record displayed is the client's medical record and if not, select the correct client from the list of clients.

_____ 2. Select and prepare the medications for administration for the appropriate time period.

_____ 3. Check the client's armband and compare it with the eMAR for the client's name and medical record number.

_____ 4. Log out of the program.

_____ 5. Open the computer program for the electronic medical record and enter the user ID and password.

_____ 6. Administer the medications and document in the eMAR.

_____ 7. Access the client's eMAR.

2. A nurse is planning to witness the signature on consent forms for multiple clients being prepared for surgery. Which clients are legally able to sign a consent form giving their consent for surgery? **Select all that apply.**

1. A 16-year-old married client who is to have a Cesarean section to deliver twins
2. A 17-year-old client who needs an emergency appendectomy
3. An 88-year-old client who is fully alert and oriented but blind
4. A 59-year-old client who only speaks German
5. A 30-year-old client who just received cefuroxime (Zinicef)

1. ANSWER: 5, 1, 7, 2, 3, 6, 4.
After opening the computer program for the electronic medical record, the nurse should then enter the user ID and password. The next step should be to determine if the medical record displayed is the client's medical record and if not, select the correct client from the list of clients. The nurse should then access the client's eMAR and select and prepare the medications for administration for the appropriate time period. Next, the nurse should check the client's armband and compare it with the eMAR for the client's name and medical record number. Then administer the medications and document in the eMAR. Finally, the nurse should log out of the program.

TEST-TAKING TIP: Use step-by-step visualization to focus on the process prior to placing items in the correct order.

Content Area: Management of Care; **Category of Health Alteration:** Ethical, Legal, and Safety Issues in Nursing; **Integrated Processes:** Communication and Documentation; **Client Need:** Safe and Effective Care Environment/Management of Care/Information Technology; **Cognitive Level:** Application; **Reference:** Wilkinson, J., & Treas, L. (2011a), pp. 1007–1009. **EBP Reference:** Currell R., & Urquhart, C. (2006). Nursing record systems: Effects on nursing practice and health care outcomes. *Cochrane Library*, 2006(4): CD002099.

2. ANSWER: 1, 3, 4, 5.
A minor who is lawfully married and any competent individual 18 years of age or older can sign a surgical consent. An interpreter should be obtained for the client who only speaks German, but the client can still sign a surgical consent. Cefuroxime is an antibiotic. Clients under the influence of medications, such as narcotics, are unable to sign a consent form. A 17-year-old is a minor; the consent of a parent or guardian is required.

TEST-TAKING TIP: Because unemancipated minors may not give consent, eliminate option 2.

Content Area: Management of Care; **Category of Health Alteration:** Ethical, Legal, and Safety Issues in Nursing; **Integrated Processes:** Nursing Process Planning; **Client Need:** Safe and Effective Care Environment/Management of Care/Informed Consent; **Cognitive Level:** Application; **Reference:** Potter, P., & Perry, A. (2009), p. 333.

3. A student nurse is caring for a client on a surgical unit who is of the Jehovah's Witness faith. Which actions require a nurse, who is a preceptor for the student, to intervene? **Select all that apply.**

1. Answers a phone call in the client's room at the client's request
2. Tells a visitor who claims to be the client's relative that the client has a wound infection
3. Puts a copy of the client's history and physical (H&P) form into the student's folder for completing an assignment when returning to school
4. Informs the client that his or her hemoglobin is 7.5 mg/dL and that the client is to receive a unit of packed blood cells (PRBCs)
5. Gives the nurse his or her access code and password to the electronic medical record (EMR) so that the nurse can check the student's documentation

4. A nurse is evaluating a client's ability to correctly measure the amount of medication in a med cup. The med cup holds 30 mL and the client has stopped pouring the medication when the cup is half full. How many milliliters of medication was prepared by the client?

_____ mL. Record your answer as a whole number.

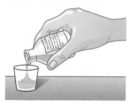

3. ANSWER: 2, 3, 4, 5.

The nurse should intervene when the student violates client confidentiality, such as in relaying protected health information (PHI) about a client without the client's consent to someone who claims to be a client's relative and taking a copy of the client's H&P record, which contains PHI. A client of the Jehovah's Witness faith will usually not accept blood or blood products. The student should not disclose an access code and password for EMRs to any other person to ensure that information about the client remains confidential. The nurse's access code and password is sufficient for the nurse to review the documentation in the client's EMR. Answering the client's telephone at the client's request does not violate client confidentiality. There is no indication that PHI is disclosed when answering the phone.

TEST-TAKING TIP: Focus on selecting options that would be considered HIPAA violations. Consider the faith beliefs of the client when reviewing options.

Content Area: Management of Care; **Category of Health Alteration:** Ethical, Legal, and Safety Issues in Nursing; **Integrated Processes:** Nursing Process Evaluation; **Client Need:** Safe and Effective Care Environment/Management of Care/Legal Rights and Responsibilities; **Cognitive Level:** Analysis; **References:** Potter, P., & Perry, A. (2009), pp. 406–408, 457. Whitehead, D., Weiss, S., & Tappen, R. (2010), pp. 24–25.

4. ANSWER: 15 mL

Use a proportion formula to calculate the amount.

30 mL : 1 med cup :: X mL : $\frac{1}{2}$ med cup

X = 15 mL

TEST-TAKING TIP: Focus on what the question is asking, determining the amount in $\frac{1}{2}$ of a med cup.

Content Area: Management of Care; **Category of Health Alteration:** Ethical, Legal, and Safety Issues in Nursing; **Integrated Processes:** Nursing Process Evaluation; **Client Need:** Health Promotion and Maintenance/Principles of Teaching and Learning; **Cognitive Level:** Application; **Reference:** Potter, P., & Perry, A. (2009), pp. 696, 721–722.

5. A family member presents the card illustrated below to a nurse caring for a recently deceased client. The nurse recognizes the signature of the client on the line for the signature of a donor. Which initial intervention is best based on the information on the card?

UNIFORM DONOR CARD SIDE 1	UNIFORM DONOR CARD SIDE 2
Marilyn Brown	Signed by the donor and two witnesses in the presence of each other
Print or type name of donor	
	Marilyn Brown 9/9/50
If medically acceptable upon my death, I hereby make this anatomical gift in the hope that I may help others. The words and marks below indicate my desires, to take effect upon my death. I wish to donate the organs or body parts designated for the purpose of transplantation, therapy, medical research or education:	Signature of donor Donor DOB
	7-17-2009 Minneapolis, MN
	Date signed City and State
	David Green *Roberta Smith*
	Witness Witness
	This is a legal document under the Uniform Anatomical Gift Act.
1) **NO** any needed organs or body parts	
2) **YES** only the following organs or body parts:	**Clearview Transplant Program**
	800-Donors-1
Skin tissue only	1234 Case Street
Specify the organ(s) or body part(s)	Minneapolis, MN 56303
3) **NO** my body for anatomical study if needed.	
4) **NO** limitations of specific wishes, if any:	

1. Call the procurement agency to inform them that the client bearing the card has recently died.
2. Notify the health care provider (HCP) and nursing supervisor of the deceased client's wishes to donate organs or body parts.
3. Ask the family about the possibility of donating the deceased client's liver and kidneys.
4. Obtain an autopsy order from the HCP so that the client's body can be donated for anatomical study.

5. ANSWER: 2.
**Agency policy and procedure should be followed as to who should con-
tact the organ procurement agency. Both the HCP and nursing supervisor
should be notified because the body needs to be released to the procurement agency.** Calling the procurement agency is premature and should be
done by the appropriate health care personnel. The wishes of the client for
organ donation only included the skin and not the liver and kidneys. An
autopsy prior to organ procurement is unnecessary. An autopsy may be
performed at the request of the family or if the death meets certain criteria, such as suspected murder or suicide.

TEST-TAKING TIP: The key word is "initial." If uncertain, think about your
actions in situations of uncertainty.

Content Area: Management of Care; **Category of Health Alteration:** Ethical, Legal,
and Safety Issues in Nursing; **Integrated Processes:** Nursing Process Implementation;
Client Need: Safe and Effective Care Environment/Management of Care/Advocacy;
Cognitive Level: Analysis; **Reference:** Craven, R., & Hirnle, C. (2009), p. 92.

6. A nurse working in the emergency department is admitting four clients involved in a motor vehicle accident who are found to have the skin conditions illustrated. For which client with the skin condition illustrated should the nurse anticipate information would be reported and disclosed to authorized public health officials? Place an X on the skin condition that should be disclosed to public health officials.

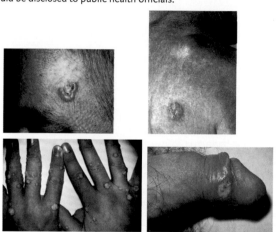

6. ANSWER: X

The illustration shows a syphilis chancre. The Health Insurance Portability and Accountability Act (HIPAA) privacy rule permits use and disclosure of protected health information (PHI) without an individual's authorization or permission for preventing or controlling disease.

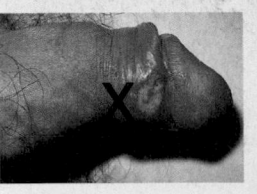

Agency policies for reporting communicable diseases must be followed and client confidentiality maintained. A nurse is ethically and legally obligated to keep information about clients confidential. The other illustrations show skin conditions that are not required to be reported. The first illustration is a basal cell carcinoma, the second an epidermoid cyst, and the third illustration is of warts.

TEST-TAKING TIP: Select an illustration that shows a communicable disease.

Content Area: Management of Care; **Category of Health Alteration:** Ethical, Legal, and Safety Issues in Nursing; **Integrated Processes:** Nursing Process Planning; **Client Need:** Safe and Effective Care Environment/Management of Care/Legal Rights and Responsibilities; **Cognitive Level:** Analysis; **Reference:** Potter, P., & Perry, A. (2009). p. 385; **EBP Reference:** United States Department of Health & Human Services (2003). *Summary of the HIPAA Privacy Rule.* Retrieved from: www.hhs.gov/ocr/privacy/hipaa/understanding/summary/privacysummary.pdf

7. A health care provider (HCP) writes the orders exhibited. A nurse reviewing the orders determines that the HCP needs to be consulted to clarify the orders. How many of the orders should the nurse clarify with the health care provider?

_____ orders. Record your answer as a whole number.

ORDER SHEET

Date	Time	
5-9-2011	1600	1. Check serum K level now.
		2. Administer 10 mEq KCL in 100 mL NaCl if potassium level is less than 3.2 mEq/L.
		3. Oxygen 2–4 L/NC.
		4. Infuse 1 liter of 0.9% NaCl with 20 mEq KCL intravenously at 100 mL per hour.
		5. Obtain surgical consent for BKA.
		6. NPO Ø meds.

8. At 0200 hours a health care provider (HCP) prescribes one unit of packed red blood cells (PRBCs) now and a hemoglobin (Hgb) level drawn at 0700. At 0730 a nurse is told at morning report that the blood is not yet available for administration. When the day shift nurse calls the blood bank, the nurse learns that the PRBCs have been ready since 0400 and that the night shift nurse was notified. Prioritize the nurse's actions by placing each step in the correct numerical order (1–6).

_____ 1. Review the client's Hgb level drawn at 0700.

_____ 2. Complete a variance report.

_____ 3. Notify the HCP of the findings and that the PRBCs were not administered.

_____ 4. Document notifying the HCP and initiate any new orders received.

_____ 5. Assess the client's vital signs and complete a focused assessment.

_____ 6. Evaluate client response to interventions.

7. ANSWER: 3

The route in order number 2 is missing for administering the 10 mEq KCL. In order number 5, the side of the body is not indicated, and although BKA commonly refers to below the knee amputation, abbreviations should not be used on a surgical consent form. In order number 6, NPO Ø meds could be misinterpreted as NPO no meds or NPO for except meds. The remaining orders are correctly written using acceptable and commonly recognized abbreviations.

TEST-TAKING TIP: Carefully read the orders. Question any order that is incomplete (route or site missing) or uses abbreviations that are unclear.

Content Area: Management of Care; **Category of Health Alteration:** Ethical, Legal, and Safety Issues in Nursing; **Integrated Processes:** Nursing Process Evaluation; **Client Need:** Safe and Effective Care Environment/Safety and Infection Control/ Error Prevention; **Cognitive Level:** Analysis; **Reference:** Berman, A., Snyder, S., & McKinney, D. (2011), p. 199.

8. ANSWER: 5, 1, 3, 4, 6, 2.

First, assess the client's vital signs and complete a focused assessment to determine the client's status. Next, review the client's hemoglobin level drawn at 0700. Then, notify the HCP of the findings and that the PRBCs were not yet administered. Document notifying the HCP and initiate any new orders received. Depending on the client's status and Hgb level, new orders might include additional PRBCs, a different blood product, or holding the PRBCs. Evaluate the client's response to the interventions. Finally, complete a variance report because the HCP's orders were not implemented.

TEST-TAKING TIP: Use the steps of the nursing process (assessment, analysis, planning, implementation, and evaluation) to place items in the correct order.

Content Area: Management of Care; **Category of Health Alteration:** Ethical, Legal and Safe Issues in Nursing; **Integrated Processes:** Nursing Process Implementation; **Client Need:** Safe and Effective Care Environment/Safety and Infection Control/ Reporting of Incident/Event/Irregular Occurrence/Variance; **Cognitive Level:** Analysis; **Reference:** Potter, P., & Perry, A. (2009), pp. 319–321.

9. A client is admitted with new onset atrial fibrillation. A new nurse on orientation receives the laboratory report illustrated for the client at 0600 hours. The nurse is uncertain about what to do next. Which actions should be taken by the new nurse? **Select all that apply.**

SERUM LABORATORY REPORT: CLIENT VALUES

Cr 1.0 mg/dL
Glucose 70 mg/dL
K 3.1 mEq/L

1. Consult the mentor to learn what actions to take.
2. Wait until morning rounds to notify the health care provider (HCP) of the normal laboratory test results.
3. Consult the charge nurse about the next steps related to the high serum creatinine level.
4. Consult the pharmacist to determine how glucagon (Glucogen) should be administered.
5. Review the HCP's orders for a protocol or order related to potassium results.

10. A nurse is working on a hospital nursing unit. Which actions by the nurse demonstrate ethical practice? **Select all that apply.**

1. Notifies a health care provider about a client who refuses to go for dialysis treatments and wants to discontinue them.
2. Informs the nurse manager of the inability to stay overtime for the night shift as mandated because of fatigue and then leaves at the end of the evening shift.
3. Teaches a client refusing to use an incentive spirometer about the risk of pneumonia and then encourages the client to try again.
4. States to a client, "Let's take a walk to the lounge so that your roommate can talk privately to her health care provider about the results of her breast biopsy."
5. States to a client, "I don't know the answer to your question, but I will find out."
6. Confronts a coworker who is witnessed taking partial doses of medications that should be discarded for personal use and takes no further action.

9. ANSWER: 1, 5.

The serum potassium level is low (normal is 3.5 to 5.0 mEq/L). When a nurse lacks the knowledge to solve a problem, it is appropriate to consult with a more experienced nurse, such as the mentor. The nurse should review HCP orders to determine if there is a protocol relating to low potassium levels. The serum laboratory results are abnormal and the HCP should be notified. Waiting until later in the morning to contact the HCP will result in a delay of necessary client treatment and is inappropriate. The low serum potassium can cause cardiac dysrhythmias, such as the atrial fibrillation. The pharmacist may be consulted to learn about potassium supplements but it is unnecessary to ask about glucagon because the client is not hypoglycemic. Normal serum glucose levels are 70 to 110 mg/dL.

TEST-TAKING TIP: Note that only the serum potassium level is low. Eliminate options that would delay client treatment. Select options that would help ensure that the nurse adheres to the accepted standard of care.

Content Area: Management of Care; **Category of Health Alteration:** Ethical, Legal, and Safety Issues in Nursing; **Integrated Processes:** Nursing Process Analysis; **Client Need:** Safe and Effective Care Environment/Management of Care/Collaboration with Interdisciplinary Team; **Cognitive Level:** Application; **References:** Berman, A., Snyder, S., & McKinney, D. (2011), pp. 169, 179, 207. Whitehead, D., Weiss, S., & Tappen, R. (2010), pp. 26–29, 80.

10. ANSWER: 1, 3, 5.

Option 1 demonstrates respect for client autonomy in refusing treatment. Option 3 demonstrates beneficence which is doing what is best for the client. Option 5 demonstrates veracity (truth telling). Option 2 demonstrates insubordination and client abandonment. Option 4 violates client confidentiality by disclosing that the roommate had a breast biopsy. Option 6 demonstrates unethical practice. Most employers have policies that encourage the reporting of witnessed theft or unprofessional conduct.

TEST-TAKING TIP: Select options that demonstrate client autonomy, beneficence, and veracity.

Content Area: Management of Care; **Category of Health Alteration:** Ethical, Legal, and Safety Issues in Nursing; **Integrated Processes:** Nursing Process Implementation; **Client Need:** Safe and Effective Care Environment/Management of Care/Ethical Practice; **Cognitive Level:** Analysis; **References:** Potter, P., & Perry, A. (2009), pp. 314–315, 335. Whitehead, D., Weiss, S., & Tappen, R. (2010), pp. 186, 188–189.

Test 2: Management of Care: Leadership and Management

11. A nurse is caring for a client on the telemetry unit who is expecting to be discharged, but discharge orders have not yet been received. After telephoning the health care provider (HCP), the nurse relays to the client that the HCP will see the client in 40 minutes. The client demands to see the Medical Director now. Which actions by the nurse are most appropriate? **Select all that apply.**

1. Contact the HCP's supervisor.
2. Report the situation immediately to the charge nurse.
3. Contact the Medical Director.
4. Apologize for the delay.
5. Inform the client that a discharge order is needed before proceeding further.
6. Clarify the client's concerns.

12. A nurse is calling a health care provider (HCP) about treatments prescribed for a client and the client's status. In which sequence should the nurse make the following statements to the HCP using the SBAR (situation, background, assessment, recommendation) communication model? Place each statement in the correct numerical order (1–4).

_____ 1. Mr. Brown, 64 years old, had a total right knee replacement 2 days ago. He also has a history of chronic atrial fibrillation.

_____ 2. Mr. Brown is due to receive warfarin (Coumadin) 5 mg orally and his international normalized ratio (INR) is 4.0.

_____ 3. Do you want me to hold the dose of warfarin? Are there any other orders you would like implemented?

_____ 4. Mr. Brown's blood pressure is 120/80, his heart rate is 90 and irregular, and high right knee dressing is clean, dry, and intact. There are no signs of active bleeding.

11. ANSWER: 2, 4.
The nurse should follow the chain of command to report problems or concerns. The nurse's immediate supervisor is the charge nurse. The nurse should use communication skills with an angry client to defuse the situation before it escalates. Offering an apology and showing interest in the client may help to defuse the situation. Contacting the HCP's supervisor or the Medical Director would not be following the chain of command. Informing the client that a discharge order is needed before proceeding further does not address the issue or the client's demand to see the Medical Director, and could escalate the problem.

TEST-TAKING TIP: Select the options that follow the nurse's chain of command and that may help to defuse the situation.

Content Area: Management of Care; **Category of Health Alteration:** Leadership and Management; **Integrated Processes:** Caring; Nursing Process Implementation; **Client Need:** Safe and Effective Care Environment/Management of Care/Concepts of Management; **Cognitive Level:** Application; **References:** Marquis, B. L., & Huston, C. J. (2009), p. 448. Whitehead, D., Weiss, S., & Tappen, R. (2010), p. 81.

12. ANSWER: 2, 1, 4, 3.
The sequence of the communication using the SBAR model should be first the statement about the situation: Mr. Brown is due to receive warfarin (Coumadin) 5 mg orally and his international normalized ratio (INR) is 4.0. The second statement should be the background: Mr. Brown, 64 years old, had a total right knee replacement 2 days ago. He also has a history of chronic atrial fibrillation. The third statement is the assessment: Mr. Brown's blood pressure is 120/80, his heart rate is 90 and irregular, and high right knee dressing is clean, dry, and intact. There are no signs of active bleeding. The last statements are the recommendation: Do you want me to hold the dose of warfarin? Are there any other orders you would like implemented?

TEST-TAKING TIP: Use the descriptions for the SBAR acronym as a guide in placing the statements in the correct sequence. The SBAR provides a framework for communicating critical client information to improve client safety.

Content Area: Management of Care; **Category of Health Alteration:** Leadership and Management; **Integrated Processes:** Communication and Documentation; **Client Need:** Safe and Effective Care Environment/Management of Care/Consultation; **Cognitive Level:** Application; **Reference:** Whitehead, D., Weiss, S., & Tappen, R. (2010), pp. 80–81.

13. Several nurses working on a medical unit are unhappy about the use of multiple protocols that place increased demands on nurses time and seemingly increase the number of errors. Which statements, if made by a nursing staff member, suggest a unit culture characteristic of transformational leadership? **Select all that apply.**

1. "When I discussed this concern with our nurse manager, the nurse manager suggested that I place this on the weekly staff meeting agenda so we can get staff input."
2. "I discussed the use of the protocols with our nurse manager and the nurse manager will take this concern to the Medical Director."
3. "I talked to the charge nurse who told me that this concern is already being addressed by management."
4. "The charge nurse has made a list of the actual errors from using the protocols and told me we can send these specifics to the nurse manager and Medical Director."
5. "We should discuss the use of protocols with our nurse educator to see if there are some strategies we could use to help us better implement the protocols."

14. A staff nurse observes the action illustrated being performed on the client who had a posterior cervical laminectomy the previous day. Which should be the staff nurse's **next** action?

1. Hand the coworker a mask for performing rescue breathing.
2. Check hand placement for compressions and be ready to begin compressions after two breaths are delivered.
3. Inform the coworker that a jaw thrust maneuver should be used to open the client's airway.
4. Activate the agency's emergency response system.

13. ANSWER: 1, 5.
Transformational leaders engage all members of the health care team to identify and solve problems. Gaining input from all stakeholders by discussion at a regularly scheduled meeting is an integral step for collaborative problem identification and problem solving. A transformational leader will encourage everyone to speak and build consensus as to what the exact problem is and how it should be solved within the organizational unit goals. Transformational leadership also involves factors such as creativity and inspiration. Taking a concern to the Medical Director or the charge nurse without staff input to identify and solve a problem is an example of using the chain of command to solve problems, but this action does not empower staff.

TEST-TAKING TIP: Focus on the statement that empowers the nurse's to seek a resolution to the problem. Note that three options have a similar action and two options are different.

Content Area: Management of Care; **Category of Health Alteration:** Leadership and Management; **Integrated Processes:** Communication and Documentation; **Client Need:** Safe and Effective Care Environment/Management of Care/Concepts of Management; **Cognitive Level:** Application; **Reference:** Marquis, B. L., & Huston, C. J. (2009), pp. 42–44.

14. ANSWER: 3.
The jaw thrust maneuver should be used and the responding nurse should correct the coworker to prevent injury to the surgical area and possible compression of the spinal cord. Although readying a mask, performing chest compression, and activating the emergency response system are appropriate actions, these are not the next action.

TEST-TAKING TIP: Select the option that would prevent further harm to the client.

Content Area: Management of Care; **Category of Health Alteration:** Ethical, Legal, and Safety Issues in Nursing; **Integrated Processes:** Nursing Process Implementation; **Client Need:** Safe and Effective Care Environment/Management of Care/Supervision; Physiological Integrity/Physiological Adaptation/Medical Emergencies; **Cognitive Level:** Analysis; **Reference:** Myers, E., & Hopkins, T. (2008), p. 167.

15. A client has an intravenous (IV) solution infusing. During the middle of a shift, a nurse enters the assigned client's room and observes another nurse performing the action illustrated. Which should be the **initial** action by the nurse making the observation?

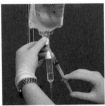

1. Ask why the nurse is injecting medication into the client's IV bag.
2. Clamp the client's running IV line.
3. Report the nurse's actions to the nurse manager.
4. Complete a variance report.

16. A nurse is rearranging room assignments for several hospitalized clients to accommodate a newly admitted client. Which clients should the nurse assign to the same room? **Select all that apply.**

1. A 32-year-old female second day postoperative cholecystectomy and a 40-year-old female with pain due to pancreatitis
2. A 36-year-old female with diarrhea and vomiting of unknown etiology and a 37-year-old female client receiving chemotherapy for colon cancer
3. An 82-year-old male who has pneumonia and candidiasis in the groin skin folds and a 76-year-old male who has an upper respiratory tract infection and thrush
4. A 46-year-old male with a *MRSA* infection and a 50-year-old with a *C. difficile* infection
5. An 18-year-old female one day postoperative appendectomy and an 84-year-old female who is agitated and confused

15. ANSWER: 2.

Because it appears that another nurse is injecting a medication or substance into the client's IV bag, the nurse should first clamp the client's running IV line to protect the client from receiving the medication or substance being injected. Although the nurse's actions should be questioned and reported to the nurse manager, and a variance report completed, these actions are not the priority. The nurse manager should be questioning the nurse's actions, gathering additional information, and evaluating for professional negligence, malpractice, or impairment issues.

TEST-TAKING TIP: The key word is "initial." Select the option that addresses client safety.

Content Area: Management of Care; **Category of Health Alteration:** Leadership and Management; **Integrated Processes:** Nursing Process Implementation; **Client Need:** Safe and Effective Care Environment/Management of Care/Legal Rights and Responsibilities; **Cognitive Level:** Analysis; **References:** Marquis, B. L., & Huston, C. J. (2009), pp. 98–99. Whitehead, D., Weiss, S., & Tappen, R. (2010), pp. 185–188.

16. ANSWER: 1, 3.

Both clients in option 1 would need frequent pain assessment and pain management interventions. Both clients in option 3 have similar respiratory conditions. Candidiasis and thrush (oral candidiasis) are fungal infections from the same causative microorganism. A client receiving chemotherapy will be immunocompromised and should not be placed with a client with diarrhea. Although the clients with *MRSA* and *C. difficile* infections will both require contact isolation, the causative organisms are different. The developmental needs of the clients in option 5 are too diverse. The 18-year-old will likely have multiple visitors that could increase the older adult client's agitation and confusion.

TEST-TAKING TIP: Select only the options in which clients have similar needs or similar conditions and eliminate other options.

Content Area: Management of Care; **Category of Health Alteration:** Leadership and Management; **Integrated Processes:** Nursing Process Planning; **Client Need:** Safe and Effective Care Environment/Management of Care/Continuity of Care; **Cognitive Level:** Analysis; **Reference:** Potter, P., & Perry, A. (2009), p. 663.

17. An experienced nurse is reviewing a new nurse's documentation in a client's medical record. Which abbreviation should the experienced nurse ask the new nurse to correct because it is on the "Do Not Use" list issued by the Joint Commission? Place an X on the **unapproved** abbreviation.

PROGRESS NOTES

Date	Time	Entry
3-20-11	1400	4 mg morphine sulfate administered IV for chest pain (CP) rated at 9 out of 10 at 1330. Within 5 minutes, CP rated at 1. No further episodes of CP. Currently has ringing in A.S. after furosemide 40 mg IV push given. Dr. Brown notified _____J. Green, RN

18. A nurse manager counsels a nurse on improving organizational skills and efficient use of time in providing safe care to clients. Which actions demonstrate that the nurse has improved in these abilities? **Select all that apply.**

1. Prepares all medications for assigned clients, places them all on one tray, and then delivers the medications to each client
2. Asks a client about her feelings related to the loss of her spouse while collecting the client's urine specimen
3. Teaches a client about using the incentive spirometer immediately after assessing the client's lung sounds
4. Obtains exam gloves, sterile gloves, a sterile dressing, tape, and a bio-hazard bag prior to entering a client's room to perform a dressing change
5. Asks an x-ray technician who enters the room to take a chest film for suspected pneumonia to return later because the nurse is about to give the client a bath

17. ANSWER: X

3-20-11   1400

4 mg morphine sulfate administered IV for chest pain (CP) rated at 9 out of 10 at 1330. Within 5 minutes, CP rated at 1. No further episodes of

| **X** |

CP. Currently has ringing in A.S. after furosemide 40 mg IV push given. Dr. Brown notified _____

_____J. Green, RN

A.S. (left ear) can be mistaken for OS (left eye), OD (right eye), or OU (both eyes).

TEST-TAKING TIP: Recall the abbreviations on the "Do Not Use" list by the Joint Commission.

Content Area: Management of Care; **Category of Health Alteration:** Leadership and Management; **Integrated Processes:** Communication and Documentation; **Client Need:** Safe and Effective Care Environment/Management of Care/Supervision; **Cognitive Level:** Analysis; **Reference:** Berman, A., Snyder, S., & McKinney, D. (2011), pp. 198–199.

18. ANSWER: 3, 4.
Efficiency includes both combining nursing activities and doing things correctly. Assessment and teaching can be combined to increase efficiency. Having all necessary supplies demonstrates organization. It is unsafe to prepare medications for all clients and then distribute them because one client's medications could be accidentally administered to another client. Asking about a client's feelings on a sensitive topic unrelated to an activity that may be embarrassing is inappropriate. The need for the chest film in treating the client is more important than giving the client a bath.

TEST-TAKING TIP: Eliminate any options that unsafely combine nursing activities, use inappropriate communication techniques, or delay a client's diagnosis.

Content Area: Management of Care; **Category of Health Alteration:** Leadership and Management; **Integrated Processes:** Nursing Process Evaluation; **Client Need:** Safe and Effective Care Environment/Management of Care/Supervision; **Cognitive Level:** Analysis; **Reference:** Potter, P., & Perry, A. (2009), pp. 307–308.

Test 3: Management of Care: Prioritization and Delegation

19. A nursing assistant (NA) employed at a hospital is working under the direction of a nurse. The NA is in the third year of a registered nurse program and has been administering medications and performing procedures during clinical experience as a student nurse. Which actions describe appropriate delegation to the NA by the nurse? **Select all that apply.**

1. Asks the NA to prepare oral medications for a stable client
2. Asks the NA to witness a client's consent prior to surgery.
3. Asks the NA to write the amounts a client has eaten on the menu and post it confidentially outside the client's door.
4. Asks the NA to complete an independent check of a dose the RN prepared to administer in an insulin pen.
5. Ask the NA to secure a wheelchair and take a client for a chest x-ray.

20. In assessing a client who sustained chest injuries in a motor vehicle accident, a nurse finds the client's respiratory rate to be 40 breaths per minute, breath sounds absent on the right side with auscultation, and the trachea deviated to the left. In which order should the nurse implement actions to care for the client? Place each action in the correct numerical order (1–4).

_____ 1. Call the patient care assistant (PCA) to bring a large-bore needle, a chest tube insertion set-up kit, and a water seal drainage system and place these at the client's bedside.
_____ 2. Notify the health care provider (HCP).
_____ 3. Ask another nurse to monitor the client.
_____ 4. Discuss the situation with the client's spouse who just arrived.

19. ANSWER: 3, 5.
A student nurse, while working as an employee of a facility, is only allowed to perform tasks listed in the job description of a NA. Legally, the NA must perform within the job description even though the NA has received instruction and acquired competence as a nursing student. The NA can post a client's menu after recording the amounts eaten, obtain supplies, and transport clients. A nursing assistant's job description would not include preparing and double-checking medications, and witnessing a client's consent.

TEST-TAKING TIP: The issue of the question is the tasks that the nurse can legally delegate to a NA who is also a student nurse. Select tasks within a typical NA job description.

Content Area: Management of Care; **Category of Health Alteration:** Prioritization and Delegation; **Integrated Processes:** Nursing Process Planning; **Client Need:** Safe and Effective Care Environment/Management of Care/Delegation; **Cognitive Level:** Analysis; **Reference:** Berman, A., Snyder, S., & McKinney, D. (2011), pp. 358–359.

20. ANSWER: 3, 2, 1, 4.
The client's absent breath sounds on the right side, tachypnea, and deviation of the trachea to the left side indicates that the client possibly has a tension pneumothorax. Continuous client monitoring is priority while the nurse next notifies the HCP. Because immediate intervention is necessary with a tension pneumothorax, the next priority is having the equipment at the bedside. A large-bore needle will be inserted by the HCP into the second intercostal space in the midclavicular line of the affected side as initial treatment. Then a chest tube is placed into the fourth intercostal space and is attached to a water seal drainage system until the lung reinflates. Finally, the nurse should discuss the situation with the client's spouse.

TEST-TAKING TIP: Focus on the key words "chest injuries in a motor vehicle accident" and secondarily on the assessed parameters. Use the ABCs (airway, breathing, circulation) to place the options in order of priority. Remember, the client is the first priority.

Content Area: Management of Care; **Category of Health Alteration:** Prioritization and Delegation; **Integrated Processes:** Nursing Process Implementation; **Client Need:** Safe and Effective Care Environment/Management of Care/Establishing Priorities; **Cognitive Level:** Application; **Reference:** Ignatavicius, D., & Workman, M. (2010), p. 699.

21. A nurse is caring for a client when the client becomes unresponsive and has the cardiac rhythm illustrated. After activating the emergency response system, which action should be taken by the nurse?

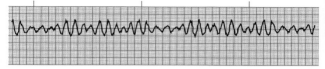

1. Applying defibrillator pads and administering a shock
2. Giving 30 chest compressions
3. Giving two rescue breaths prior to starting chest compressions
4. Checking for the client's carotid pulse

22. A client has a gastrostomy tube in place and needs assistance with personal care, toileting, and feeding. When considering delegation of aspects of the client's care, which components of delegation should a nurse consider? **Select all that apply.**

1. Right person
2. Right task
3. Right health care provider (HCP)
4. Right circumstances
5. Right supervision
6. Right direction/communication

21. ANSWER: 1.
The client's rhythm is ventricular fibrillation. Defibrillation should occur as soon as possible to convert the client's rhythm. Although chest compressions, rescue breathing, and checking for the client's carotid pulse are all aspects of CPR, these activities should not delay the use of a defibrillator, which is needed to attempt to convert the client's rhythm.

TEST-TAKING TIP: Use word association to remember the action that is most important: "treat ventricular fibrillation with defibrillation."

Content Area: Management of Care; **Category of Health Alteration:** Prioritization and Delegation; **Integrated Processes:** Nursing Process Implementation; **Client Need:** Safe and Effective Care Environment/Management of Care/ Establishing Priorities; **Cognitive Level:** Application; **Reference:** Ignatavicius, D., & Workman, M. (2010), pp. 748–750.

22. ANSWER: 1, 2, 4, 5, 6.
The five rights of delegation include the right task, right circumstances, right person, right direction/communication, and right supervision/ evaluation. The right HCP is rarely part of delegation, as most delegation does not involve a HCP.

TEST-TAKING TIP: There are "five" rights of delegation, so only five options are correct.

Content Area: Management of Care; **Category of Health Alteration:** Prioritization and Delegation; **Integrated Processes:** Nursing Process Planning; **Client Need:** Safe and Effective Care Environment/Management of Care/Delegation; **Cognitive Level:** Application; **Reference:** Whitehead, D., Weiss, S., & Tappen, R. (2010), p. 117.

23. A nurse receives shift report at 0700 on four pediatric clients. In which order should the nurse assess the clients? Place the order in which the nurse should assess these children in the correct numerical sequence (1–4).

_____ 1. A 3-year-old who is crying because a parent just left
_____ 2. A 1-year-old with a blood pressure (BP) of 94/50
_____ 3. A 2-year-old weighing 15 kg whose IV has been infusing at 20 mL/kg/hr for the past 4 hr
_____ 4. A 4-year-old with a blood glucose level of 59 mg/dL

24. A nurse is caring for multiple clients on a hospital nursing unit. Which actions should the nurse plan to delegate to an unlicensed ancillary personnel (UAP)? **Select all that apply.**

1. Applying a warm compress to a client's arm to enhance vein distention
2. Instilling artificial tears eye drops to a client experiencing dry eyes
3. Teaching a client with pneumonia about the importance of adequate fluid intake
4. Reminding a client to use an incentive spirometer (IS) every 1 to 2 hours while awake
5. Transferring a client from the bed to a chair prior to a meal

23. ANSWER: 3, 4, 1, 2.
A 2-year-old weighing 15 kg whose IV has been infusing at 20 mL/kg/hr
for the past 4 hr has been receiving IV fluids at 300 mL/hr. The child is at
risk for fluid volume overload if this rate is correct. The next client for the
nurse to assess is the 4-year-old with a blood glucose level of 59 mg/dL.
The normal range is 60–100 mg/dL for a child, and the value is slightly
low. The child who is crying should be assessed third because the child
needs to be comforted. The last child to be assessed should be the
1-year-old who has a BP within the normal range for the age of the child.

TEST-TAKING TIP: Use the ABCs (airway, breathing, circulation) to establish priority. Because no options deal with airway, examine the options that
affect circulation. Consider whether the IV infusion rate is appropriate and
whether the blood pressure is normal. The client with normal findings
should be assessed last. Remember that the normal blood glucose range
for a 4-year-old child is 10 mg/dL lower than for an adult.

Content Area: Management of Care; **Category of Health Alteration:** Prioritization
and Delegation; **Integrated Processes:** Nursing Process Planning; **Client Need:** Safe
and Effective Care Environment/Management of Care/Establishing Priorities;
Cognitive Level: Analysis; **Reference:** Ball, J., & Bindler, R. (2008), p. 510.

24. ANSWER: 1, 4, 5.
The scope of practice for UAPs includes assisting with basic care, such as
applying a warm compress, reminders to use the IS, which is already a
part of the plan of care, and positioning. It does not include medication
administration and client teaching, both of which require additional education and skill and are within the RN scope of practice.

TEST-TAKING TIP: Eliminate options that would require additional education and skill.

Content Area: Management of Care; **Category of Health Alteration:** Prioritization
and Delegation; **Integrated Processes:** Nursing Process Planning; **Client Need:** Safe
and Effective Care Environment/Management of Care/Delegation; **Cognitive Level:**
Analysis; **Reference:** Berman, A., Snyder, S., & McKinney, D. (2011), pp. 358–359.

25. A nurse assesses the pupil size of a client who has an epidural hematoma. Following the assessment, the nurse immediately notifies the health care provider (HCP) thinking that the client may have increased intracranial pressure with compression of the oculomotor nerve. Place an X on the pupil size that would **best** support the nurse's conclusion?

Pupil gauge (mm)

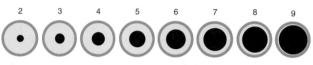

2 3 4 5 6 7 8 9

26. A nurse administers hydromorphone (Dilaudid) 2 mg IV to a postoperative client. Thirty minutes later the client states to the nurse, "I don't know why the medication hasn't taken effect. I'm still hurting. I'm worried that something's wrong." Which actions should be taken by the nurse? **Select all that apply.**

1. Check the client for bladder distention.
2. Insert a nasogastric tube for stomach decompression.
3. Determine the time of the client's last void.
4. Call the health care provider (HCP) for an increase in medication dose.
5. Reassure the client that it may take more time for the medication dose to be effective.

25. ANSWER:

Pupil gauge (mm)

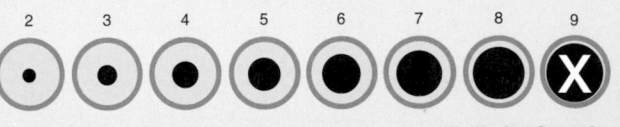

2 3 4 5 6 7 8 9

Compression of the oculomotor nerve results in pupil dilation from the shifting of the brain and paralyzing the muscles controlling pupillary size and shape. It is a neurological emergency that indicates herniation of the brain.

TEST-TAKING TIP: If unsure, select the largest pupil size because the oculomotor nerve controls the muscles of the eye and this is compressed and paralyzed.

Content Area: Management of Care; **Category of Health Alteration:** Prioritization and Delegation; **Integrated Processes:** Nursing Process Assessment; **Client Need:** Safe and Effective Care Environment/Management of Care/Establishing Priorities; **Cognitive Level:** Application; **Reference:** Black, J. & Hawks, J. (2009), 1923, 1929–1931.

26. ANSWER: 1, 3.
The nurse should assess for bladder distention and determine the time of the client's last void because bladder atony can occur after an inguinal herniorrhaphy and a full bladder can cause pain. There is no indication that the client has abdominal distention, nausea, or vomiting; inserting a nasogastric tube is unnecessary. Calling the HCP is premature. Although reassurance is important to reduce the client's anxiety, the onset of hydromorphone administered IV is 15 minutes with a peak effect in 30 to 90 minutes.

TEST-TAKING TIP: Think about the proximity of the bladder to the surgical site.

Content Area: Management of Care; **Category of Health Alteration:** Prioritization and Delegation; **Integrated Processes:** Nursing Process Implementation; **Client Need:** Safe and Effective Care Environment/Management of Care/ Establishing Priorities; **Cognitive Level:** Analysis; **Reference:** Deglin, J., Vallerand, A., & Sanoski, C. (2011), 640–642.

27. A nurse is delegating to a nursing assistant (NA) initiating a 24-hour urine collection for a client. Which statements demonstrate appropriate delegation? **Select all that apply.**

1. "Put a container in the client's bathroom for collecting the urine."
2. "Ensure that all urine is transferred to the container and kept on ice."
3. "Remind the client to save all urine with each voiding."
4. "Explain the purpose of the 24-hour urine collection to the client."
5. "Record the amount the client voids on the intake and output record."
6. "Document the color, odor, and whether or not there is sediment in the client's urine."

28. A nurse enters the hospital room of a 5-year-old child who is choking. Place each step in the correct numerical order (1–6) for treating the child who becomes unresponsive after the nurse performs abdominal thrusts.

_____ 1. Straddle the child.
_____ 2. Give five quick firm thrusts inward and upward and then check the child's mouth.
_____ 3. Give a rescue breath.
_____ 4. Lower the child to the floor.
_____ 5. Check the child's mouth for the object.
_____ 6. Place the heel of one hand with other hand over it in the middle of the child's abdomen just above the umbilicus.

27. ANSWER: 1, 2, 3, 5.
Obtaining supplies, transferring urine into a container on ice, reminding the client about saving the urine, and recording output are within the scope of practice of a NA. Teaching and assessment are functions within the RN scope of practice and cannot be delegated.

TEST-TAKING TIP: Eliminate options that require additional education and are within the professional nurse role.

Content Area: Management of Care; **Category of Health Alteration:** Prioritization and Delegation; **Integrated Processes:** Nursing Process Evaluation; **Client Need:** Safe and Effective Care Environment/Management of Care/Delegation; **Cognitive Level:** Analysis; **Reference:** Berman, A., Snyder, S., & McKinney, D. (2011), pp. 358–359.

28. ANSWER: 4, 5, 3, 1, 6, 2.
First, lower the child to the floor, then check the child's mouth for the object. If not seen, give a quick breath. Then straddle the child and place the heel of one hand with other hand over it in the middle of the child's abdomen just above the umbilicus. Give five quick firm thrusts inward and upward and then check the child's mouth. The steps are continued until the obstruction is relieved and rescue breaths are effective.

TEST-TAKING TIP: Visualize the steps before placing these in priority order. A breath should be given before the thrust.

Content Area: Child Health; **Category of Health Alteration:** Prioritization and Delegation; **Integrated Processes:** Nursing Process Implementation; **Client Need:** Physiological Integrity/Physiological Adaptation/Medical Emergencies; **Cognitive Level:** Analysis; **Reference:** Myers, E. (2010), p. 136; **EBP Reference:** Berg, M. D., Schexnayder, S. M., Chameides, L., Terry, M., Donoghue, A., Hickey, R. W., & Hazinski, M. F. (2010). Part 13: Pediatric Basic Life Support: 2010 American Heart Association Guidelines for Cardiopulmonary Resuscitation and Emergency Cardiovascular Care, *Circulation*. 122, S862–S875, doi:10.1161/CIRCULATIONAHA.110.971085.

Test 4: Management of Care: Teaching and Learning, Communication, and Cultural Diversity

29. A nurse is adding interventions to a plan of care for a client with a nursing diagnosis of readiness for enhanced knowledge related to self blood glucose monitoring and self-administration of insulin. Which outcomes should the nurse add to the client's plan of care to best help the client achieve psychomotor learning as opposed to cognitive and affective learning? **Select all that apply.**

1. Brings own glucometer to the teaching session and imitates the nurse's actions for checking a blood glucose level.
2. Makes eye contact with the nurse as the nurse explains the process for checking a blood glucose level.
3. Explains the normal ranges for blood glucose levels.
4. Reports the names of the types of insulin being taken.
5. Measures the correct amount of insulin based on the client's blood glucose reading.

30. A nurse is evaluating whether treatment has been effective for a client diagnosed with tinea pedis. Which body areas should the nurse assess to evaluate the effectiveness of treatment? Place an X on the area the nurse should assess.

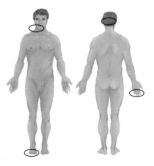

29. ANSWER: 1, 5.
Psychomotor learning includes imitation and performance of skills. Making eye contact is an affective learning behavior and, depending on the ethnicity of the client, could be culturally insensitive. Explaining and reporting are cognitive learning behaviors.

TEST-TAKING TIP: Select only the options that include motor skills.

Content Area: Management of Care; **Category of Health Alteration:** Teaching and Learning, Communication, and Cultural Diversity; **Integrated Processes:** Teaching and Learning; **Client Need:** Safe and Effective Care Environment/Management of Care/Case Management; **Cognitive Level:** Application; **Reference:** Potter, P., & Perry, A. (2009), pp. 376–383.

30. ANSWER:
Tinea pedis, athlete's foot, occurs on the soles of one or both feet with scaling and mild redness and maceration in the toe webs. The nurse should be sure to inspect between the client's toes, also.

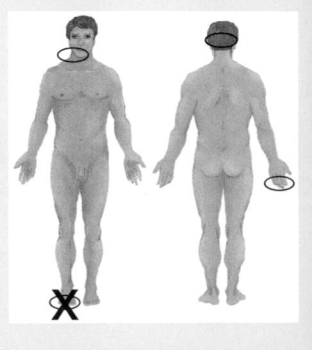

TEST-TAKING TIP: Use knowledge of medical terminology. Pedis refers to foot.

Content Area: Adult Health; **Category of Health Alteration:** Infectious Disease; **Integrated Processes:** Nursing Process Evaluation; **Client Need:** Physiological Integrity/Physiological Adaptation/Pathophysiology; **Cognitive Level:** Application; **Reference:** Smeltzer, S., Bare, B., Hinkle, J., & Cheever, K. (2010), p. 1691.

31. A child is hospitalized for treatment of acute lymphocytic leukemia and a nurse is planning time for an extensive teaching session with the child and parents. Which conditions would enhance the ability of the child and parents to comprehend the information provided by the nurse? **Select all that apply.**

1. First chemotherapy infusion has just been started.
2. Child is playing with a new toy.
3. Child rates pain at 4 out of 10 on a 0 to 10 numeric scale.
4. TV is playing in the background.
5. Soft classical background music is playing.
6. Parent is asking many questions.

32. A client, diagnosed with borderline personality disorder, is prescribed buspirone (Buspar) for anxiety. Which statements made by the client indicate that teaching has been effective? **Select all that apply.**

1. "Drinking alcohol while taking buspirone can have serious adverse effects."
2. "Even if I am feeling better I should take the medication exactly as prescribed."
3. "Before taking any over-the-counter medications I should notify the prescriber."
4. "I should avoid eating foods high in tyramine, such as aged cheese."
5. "If I plan to become pregnant, I should inform my health care provider."

31. ANSWER: 5, 6.
Research has shown that classical music is an aid to learning. Many questions by the parent indicate a readiness to learn. Anxiety limits a person's ability to retain and process information. Distraction inhibits focusing on the information. Pain limits a person's ability to retain and process information. A TV will take attention away from the lesson to be learned.

TEST-TAKING TIP: Think about situations in which you would be less likely to learn.

Content Area: Management of Care; **Category of Health Alteration:** Teaching and Learning, Communication, and Cultural Diversity; **Integrated Processes:** Teaching and Learning; **Client Need:** Health Promotion and Maintenance/Principles of Teaching and Learning; **Cognitive Level:** Application; **Reference:** Potter, P., & Perry, A. (2009), pp. 366–381.

32. ANSWER: 1, 2, 3, 5.
Alcohol, CNS depressants, and over-the-counter medications should be avoided due to the medication interactions and potentiating effects. The medication should not be abruptly discontinued. Buspirone must be discontinued during pregnancy. Foods high in tyramine do not need to be avoided. Buspirone is an anti-anxiety medication and not a monoamine oxidase inhibitor (MAOI).

TEST-TAKING TIP: If unsure, use the knowledge that buspirone is not a MAOI and there are no food restrictions to eliminate the one incorrect option.

Content Area: Management of Care; **Category of Health Alteration:** Teaching and Learning, Communication, and Cultural Diversity; **Integrated Processes:** Teaching and Learning; **Client Need:** Health Promotion and Maintenance/Principles of Teaching and Learning; **Cognitive Level:** Analysis; **Reference:** Pedersen, D. (2008), p. 130.

33. An older adult client has a stage III pressure ulcer. When teaching the client's family, a nurse identifies the layer of tissue that is damaged. Place an X on the circled area in the deepest layer of tissue that the nurse should identify as being damaged with a stage III pressure ulcer.

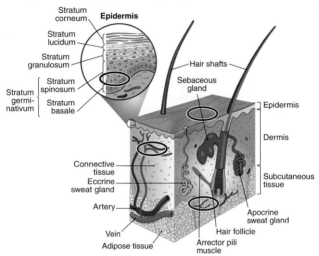

33. ANSWER:

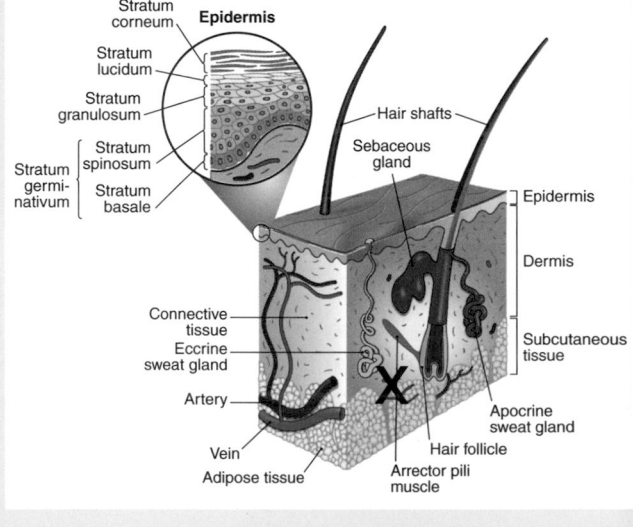

A stage III pressure ulcer involves full-thickness skin loss of dermis and epidermis and penetrates as far down as subcutaneous tissue.

TEST-TAKING TIP: Note the keywords "stage III pressure ulcer" and remember the pathophysiology of a stage III pressure ulcer extends through the first and second layer of the skin down to subcutaneous tissue.

Content Area: Management of Care; **Category of Health Alteration:** Teaching and Learning, Communication, and Cultural Diversity; **Integrated Processes:** Teaching and Learning; **Client Need:** Physiological Integrity/Physiological Adaptation/Pathophysiology; **Cognitive Level:** Analysis; **Reference:** Ignatavicius, D., & Workman, M. (2010), p. 489.

34. A nurse is assessing the spiritual and cultural needs of five clients of varying religious beliefs who are near death. Which observations should the nurse expect for the clients of the various religious faiths? **Select all that apply.**

1. The bed positioned so it is turned toward Mecca for a client of the Muslim faith
2. A priest anointing the sick and hearing the confession of a client of the Methodist faith
3. A "do-not-enter" sign posted on the room door of a male client of the Muslim faith who has just died and male family members are washing the client's body
4. A client of the Hindu faith talking with the social worker about the need for cremation within 24 hours so the client's soul is released from earthly attachments
5. A client whose ethnicity is Asian assigned to room number 444

35. A nurse is evaluating a licensed practical nurse's (LPN) ability to perform the Hemoccult screening test illustrated. The nurse determines that the LPN correctly performs the test when the nurse is observed placing which component on the window of the Hemoccult slide?

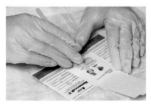

1. Urine
2. Blood
3. Stool
4. Nasal secretions

34. ANSWER: 1, 3, 4.
Muslims who are dying want their body or heads turned toward Mecca. Persons of the Muslim (Islam) faith believe in special procedures for care of the body after death, including a ritual bath with male family members washing male bodies and females washing female bodies. Persons of the Hindu faith believe in cremation within 24 hours to release the soul from any earthly attachment. A priest would anoint the sick (formerly last rites) for a person of the Catholic faith (not Methodist faith). The number or character 4 is avoided by persons of Asian ethnicity because it symbolizes death.

TEST-TAKING TIP: Focus on both the action and the faith of the client.

Content Area: Management of Care; **Category of Health Alteration:** Teaching and Learning, Communication, and Cultural Diversity; **Integrated Processes:** Nursing Process Assessment; **Client Need:** Psychosocial Integrity/Religious and Spiritual Influences on Health; Psychosocial Integrity/Cultural Diversity; **Cognitive Level:** Analysis; **References:** Berman, A., Snyder, S., Kozier, B., & Erb, G. (2008), p. 1048. Craven, R., & Hirnle, C. (2009), pp. 1401–1402. Ignatavicius, D., & Workman, M. (2010), p. 119.

35. ANSWER: 3.
Two small samples from separate areas of the client's stool should be placed on separate windows of the Hemoccult slide to perform a Hemoccult test. A urinalysis is used to test for blood in the urine. A serum laboratory test is used to test for the components in the serum, such as red blood cells (RBCs). Nasal secretions are usually not tested for the presence of blood.

TEST-TAKING TIP: If unsure, use knowledge of medical terminology to think through the answer. "Hemo-" pertains to blood. Of the options, think about the screening tests for each to test for the presence of blood.

Content Area: Management of Care; **Category of Health Alteration:** Teaching and Learning, Communication, and Cultural Diversity; **Integrated Processes:** Nursing Process Evaluation; **Client Need:** Physiological Integrity/Basic Care and Comfort/ Elimination; **Cognitive Level:** Application; **Reference:** Berman, A., Snyder, S., & McKinney, D. (2011), p. 553.

36. A client who is Hispanic tells a nurse through an interpreter that she is Roman Catholic and firmly believes in the rituals and traditions of the Catholic faith. Based on the client's statement, which actions by the nurse demonstrate cultural sensitivity and spiritual support? **Select all that apply.**

1. Administers the last rites to the client if death is imminent.
2. Offers to secure a rosary if the client states forgetting to bring items used in prayer.
3. Makes a referral for a Catholic priest to visit the client.
4. Removes the crucifix from the wall in the client's room.
5. Ensures that meals served on Friday's during Lent do not contain meat.

37. A 4-year-old client is newly diagnosed with type 1 diabetes mellitus (DM). When return-demonstrating glucose monitoring, a mother obtains the before-meal fingerstick blood glucose reading illustrated. Based on the reading, which statement to the mother is correct?

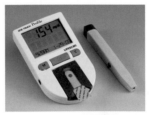

1. "Although slightly elevated, this is an acceptable before-meal value for a 4 year old."
2. "Before your child eats, administer your child's insulin to cover for this elevated reading."
3. "This is a low reading for a 4-year-old; have your child first drink a glass of juice."
4. "Your child's oral diabetic agent is effective in normalizing the blood glucose levels."

36. ANSWER: 2, 3, 5.
In times of illness, a client of the Roman Catholic faith may turn to prayer for spiritual support. This may include rosary prayers or visits from a priest who is the spiritual leader in the Roman Catholic faith. Those of the Catholic faith avoid eating meat on Fridays during Lent. A priest, not a nurse, would administer the last rites or sacrament of the sick. Members of other religious groups, such as Judaism or those with Islamic beliefs, may request that a crucifix be removed from the wall, but a crucifix is used in prayer by Catholics.

TEST-TAKING TIP: Consider the role of the spiritual leader in the Catholic faith and the spiritual symbols.

Content Area: Management of Care; **Category of Health Alteration:** Teaching and Learning, Communication, and Cultural Diversity; **Integrated Processes:** Nursing Process Implementation; **Client Need:** Psychosocial Integrity/Religious and Spiritual Influences on Health; Psychosocial Integrity/Cultural Diversity; **Cognitive Level:** Analysis; **Reference:** Harkreader, H., Hogan, M., & Thobaben, M. (2007), pp. 53; 1252–1254.

37. ANSWER: 1.
The acceptable before-meal value for a toddler with type 1 DM is 100–180 mg/dL. When the value is in the acceptable range, insulin coverage is not required. Hypoglycemia is not present; giving orange juice is unnecessary. Type 1 DM is not treated with oral agents.

TEST-TAKING TIP: The before-meal values for blood glucose are higher for toddlers and preschoolers than adults.

Content Area: Management of Care; **Category of Health Alteration:** Teaching and Learning, Communication, and Cultural Diversity; **Integrated Processes:** Teaching and Learning; **Client Need:** Physiological Integrity/Basic Care and Comfort/Nutrition and Oral Hydration; **Cognitive Level:** Analysis; **Reference:** Perry, S., Hockenberry, M., Lowdermilk, D., & Wilson, D. (2010), p. 1620.

Tab 2 **Safety and Infection Control |**
Fundamental Concepts of Nursing

Test 5: **Fundamentals:** Basic Care and Comfort

38. A nurse assesses a 3-year-old child's pain level using the Wong-Baker FACES Pain Rating Scale. When asked to point to the face, the child selects the face that is sad but not crying. At what level should a nurse document that the child rated the pain? Place an X on the number reflecting the child's pain level.

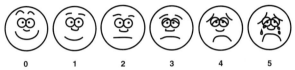

| 0 | 1 | 2 | 3 | 4 | 5 |

39. A nurse is evaluating whether a nursing assistant (NA) has correctly recorded a client's liquid intake for a shift. The client consumed 4 ounces of juice, 6 ounces of coffee, cereal, and 8 ounces of milk for breakfast. At lunch, the client ate 75% of the meat and potatoes, 100% of the vegetable, 120 mL of tea, 3 ounces of gelatin, and 8 ounces of milk. During the shift, the client drank 900 mL of water. Based on this information, how many total milliliters (mL) of liquid consumed by the client should the NA have recorded?

_____ mL (Record your answer as a whole number.)

38. ANSWER:

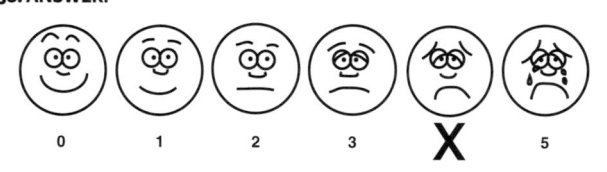

0   1   2   3   **X**   5

The value that should be recorded for the child's pain level is "4." This value reflects that the pain hurts a whole lot but not as bad as could be imagined.

TEST-TAKING TIP: Be clear about what is being asked in the question. Follow the directions carefully for hot spot items. In this question the X should be placed on the number and not the face.

Content Area: Fundamentals; **Category of Health Alteration:** Basic Care and Comfort; **Integrated Processes:** Communication and Documentation; **Client Need:** Physiological Integrity/Basic Care and Comfort/Nonpharmacological Comfort Interventions; **Cognitive Level:** Application; **Reference:** Ball, J., & Bindler, R. (2008), pp. 477–478; **EBP Reference:** Institute for Clinical Systems Improvement. (2008). *Assessment and management of acute pain.* Retrieved from www.guideline.gov/summary/summary.aspx?view_id=1&doc_id=12302.

39. ANSWER: 1890

Convert ounces to milliliters (mL). One ounce = 30 mL. Calculate only the liquid intake. Therefore, for breakfast 4 ounces juice = 120 mL, 6 ounces coffee = 180 mL, and 8 ounces milk = 240 mL. The total for breakfast is 540 mL. For lunch tea = 120 mL, 3 ounces gelatin = 90 mL, and 8 ounces of milk = 240 mL. The total for lunch is 450 mL. Add the total milliliters of fluid the client consumed during the shift (540 + 450 + 900 = 1890).

TEST-TAKING TIP: Convert ounces to milliliters to solve the problem. Be sure to use the calculator available on the NCLEX-RN examination.

Content Area: Fundamentals; **Category of Health Alteration:** Basic Care and Comfort; **Integrated Processes:** Nursing Process Evaluation; **Client Need:** Physiological Integrity/Basic Care and Comfort/Nutrition and Oral Hydration; **Cognitive Level:** Analysis; **Reference:** Berman, A., Snyder, S., Kozier, B., & Erb, G. (2008), p. 1447.

40. A client puts on the call light and a nurse finds the client lying in bed, dyspneic, and tachypneic. Which should be the initial actions by the nurse? **Select all that apply.**

1. Summon other nursing personnel for assistance.
2. Use a resuscitation bag to assist the client's breathing.
3. Assess airway patency.
4. Raise the head of the bed to high Fowler's position.
5. Monitor vital signs and oxygen saturation level.
6. Apply oxygen at 2–3 L per nasal cannula.

41. A nurse is preparing to obtain urine for a culture. Place an X at the location on one of the illustrations where the nurse should plan to obtain the urine for the specimen.

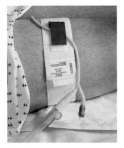 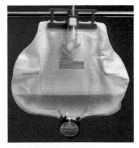

40. ANSWER: 1, 3, 4, 5, 6.
Initial nursing actions should include those that relieve the client's respiratory distress, such as obtaining help to effectively manage the situation, positioning the client to decrease breathing effort, assessing the client's condition through appropriate physical assessment, and applying oxygen. Insufficient information exists about the extent of the client's dyspnea and tachypnea. Additional information such as the respiratory rate and oxygen saturation level should be collected and other measures implemented and evaluated for effectiveness before using a resuscitation bag.

TEST-TAKING TIP: Understand that the client is in acute respiratory distress. Evaluate each option and consider how the intervention will affect the client. Eliminate option 2 because the situation in the stem does not call for use of a resuscitation bag.

Content Area: Fundamentals; **Category of Health Alteration:** Basic Care and Comfort; **Integrated Processes:** Nursing Process Implementation; **Client Need:** Physiological Integrity/Reduction of Risk Potential/Changes or Abnormalities in Vital Signs; **Cognitive Level:** Analysis; **Reference:** Potter, P., & Perry, A. (2009), p. 930.

41. ANSWER:
The sampling port on the urinary catheter should be used to collect a sterile urine specimen. The tubing should be first clamped below the sampling port, located on the side of the catheter tubing, to allow sterile urine to collect. Once collected, the urine should be obtained through the sampling port.

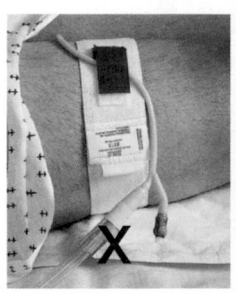

TEST-TAKING TIP: Read the item carefully. Because the urine needs to be sterile to obtain a sterile culture, eliminate the second illustration and focus on the first illustration. Differentiate the balloon inflation port from the sampling port. If unsure, look carefully at the drainage system and select the port on the drainage tubing.

Content Area: Fundamentals; **Category of Health Alteration:** Basic Care and Comfort; **Integrated Processes:** Nursing Process Planning; **Client Need:** Physiological Integrity/Basic Care and Comfort/Elimination; **Cognitive Level:** Application; **Reference:** Potter, P., & Perry, A. (2009), p. 1140.

42. Five days after a low anterior resection for colon cancer, a client is not passing flatus and has hypoactive bowel sounds. Which interventions should a nurse include in the client's plan of care? **Select all that apply.**

1. Administer bisacodyl (Dulcolax) suppository.
2. Encourage the client to expel flatus.
3. Increase opioid medication to control pain.
4. Promote frequent ambulation.
5. Encourage eating a regular diet.

43. An experienced nurse is observing a new nurse administer an intermittent gastrostomy tube feeding (TF) to a client. Which critical judgment by the experienced nurse about the new nurse's actions is **most** accurate?

1. The new nurse is exposing the client unnecessarily to administer the TF.
2. The new nurse is elevating the syringe to the correct height for an intermittent TF.
3. The new nurse should now insert the plunger of the syringe to deliver the TF.
4. The new nurse should have positioned the client flat and on the right side to administer the TF.

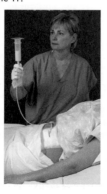

42. ANSWER: 1, 2, 4, 5.

Bisacodyl is a medication that induces peristaltic contractions by direct simulation of sensory nerve endings in the colonic wall. Some patients are hesitant to expel flatus and the nurse must provide support for this natural body activity. Ambulation stimulates contraction of intestinal smooth muscle. Eating a regular diet should be encouraged because, when food enters the stomach and duodenum, the gastrocolic and duodenocolic reflexes are initiated, resulting in peristalsis. A side effect of opioid medication is slowing of the gastrointestinal tract and constipation.

TEST-TAKING TIP: Think about the effect of opioid medications on peristalsis.

Content Area: Fundamentals; **Category of Health Alteration:** Basic Care and Comfort; **Integrated Processes:** Nursing Process Planning; **Client Need:** Physiological Integrity/Basic Care and Comfort/Elimination; **Cognitive Level:** Application; **References:** Berman, A., Snyder, S., & McKinney, D. (2011), pp. 1023–1027.

43. ANSWER: 2.

During administration of intermittent TFs, the syringe should not be elevated more than 18 inches above the insertion site. The nurse should monitor for client tolerance to the feeding, including signs of abdominal distention. Gradual emptying of the TF by gravity reduces the risk of abdominal discomfort, vomiting, or diarrhea induced by bolus or too-rapid infusion of an intermittent tube feeding. The head of the bed should be elevated for any type of TF to prevent aspiration. If the feeding is not tolerated, the client is positioned on the right side to promote stomach emptying.

TEST-TAKING TIP: Read each option carefully. Visualize the steps for administering an intermittent tube feeding to select the correct option.

Content Area: Fundamentals; **Category of Health Alteration:** Basic Care and Comfort; **Integrated Processes:** Nursing Process Analysis; **Client Need:** Physiological Integrity/Basic Care and Comfort/Nutrition and Oral Hydration; **Cognitive Level:** Analysis; **Reference:** Potter, P., & Perry, A. (2009), p. 1119.

44. A nurse uses the Braden Scale to assess and document a client's pressure sore risk. The client is slightly limited in sensory perception and is occasionally diaphoretic. The client is able to sit in a chair, but has very limited movement. The client is receiving adequate caloric intake by tube feedings, weighs 140 pounds, and has paper-thin skin but is moved easily by the nursing staff without any evidence of skin breakdown. Based on this information, which score on the Braden Scale should the nurse document in the client's medical record?

_____ score (Record your answer as a whole number.)

Criteria	Score 1	Score 2	Score 3	Score 4
Sensory perception	Completely limited	Very limited	Slightly limited	No impairment
Moisture	Constantly moist	Moist	Occasionally moist	Rarely moist
Activity	Bedfast	Chair fast	Walks occasionally	Walks frequently
Mobility	Completely immobile	Very limited	Slightly limited	No limitations
Nutrition	Very poor	Probably inadequate	Adequate	Excellent
Friction and shear	Problem	Potential problem	No apparent problem	

45. A nurse is caring for a client with arterial leg ulcers. Which recommendations for preventing complications from the leg ulcers should the nurse instruct the client to adhere to upon hospital discharge? **Select all that apply.**

1. "Avoid crossing your legs at the knees or ankles."
2. "Elevate your legs above the heart throughout the day."
3. "Massage your legs to improve circulation."
4. "Participate in regular aerobic exercises."
5. "Use moisturizing lotions for dry areas on your legs."
6. "When resting in a recliner, avoid the fully reclined position."

44. ANSWER: 15

According to the Braden Scale criteria, the client scores 3 in sensory perception, 3 in moisture, 2 in activity, 2 in mobility, 3 in nutrition, and 2 in friction and shear. The total score is 15.

TEST-TAKING TIP: Read the assessment data carefully and score each part of the Braden Scale for Predicting Pressure Sore Risk according to the chart. Add up the total of points to determine the client's score.

Content Area: Fundamentals; **Category of Health Alteration:** Basic Care and Comfort; **Integrated Processes:** Communication and Documentation; **Client Need:** Physiological Integrity/Basic Care and Comfort/Mobility/Immobility; **Cognitive Level:** Analysis; **Reference:** Potter, P., Perry, A. (2009), pp. 1288–1289.

45. ANSWER: 1, 4, 5, 6.

Crossing the legs at the knees or ankles should be avoided to prevent blood stasis. Evidence demonstrates that participation in regular aerobic exercises improves circulation to the legs. Using moisturizing lotions prevents skin breakdown. A fully reclined position in a recliner will raise the client's legs above heart level and should be avoided. The legs should be elevated no higher than the level of the heart because this would decrease circulation in the lower extremities. Vigorous massage places additional pressure on the leg vessels and can lead to an embolus if a clot is present.

TEST-TAKING TIP: Eliminate actions that will impede circulation.

Content Area: Fundamentals; **Category of Health Alteration:** Basic Care and Comfort; **Integrated Processes:** Teaching and Learning; **Client Need:** Safe and Effective Care Environment/Safety and Infection Control/Accident and Injury Prevention; **Cognitive Level:** Application; **References:** Smeltzer, S., Bare, B., Hinkle, J., & Cheever, K. (2010). p. 862.

46. A nurse is testing a client's vision by asking the client to identify numbers in the Ishihara chart illustrated. Which conclusion by a student nurse observing this test is correct?

1. The nurse is assessing the client's near-vision.
2. The nurse is assessing the client's extraocular muscular function.
3. The nurse is assessing the client's central vision.
4. The nurse is assessing the client's color vision.

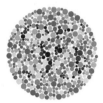

47. A nurse assesses a client who has a purulent Stage IV pressure ulcer of the sacrum that is seeping through the dressing. In which order should the nurse plan to implement measures related to care for the client's pressure ulcer? Place each step in the correct numerical order (1–6).

_____ 1. Gather all the necessary supplies to change the dressing covering the wound.

_____ 2. Premedicate the client with pain medication to reduce the pain of a dressing change.

_____ 3. Change gloves after removing the soiled dressing.

_____ 4. Wash hands and reglove before placing a sterile dressing.

_____ 5. Contain the copious amounts of purulent drainage that is seeping onto the bed linen and wash hands.

_____ 6. Wash hands, glove, and remove the soiled dressing; place in a closed bag for disposal.

46. ANSWER: 4.

The Ishihara chart tests the client's ability to recognize color. Near vision is tested by asking the client to read a Snellen card, such as the Rosenbaum Pocket Vision Screener, 14 inches from the eyes. Extraocular muscle function is assessed by observing the cardinal positions of gaze. A client with a blind spot in the central vision would have difficulty seeing the numbers if they occurred in the blind spot, but this is not the purpose of the test.

TEST-TAKING TIP: Study the diagram and note that numbers are formed from different tonal qualities of color, which points to option 4.

Content Area: Fundamentals; **Category of Health Alteration:** Basic Care and Comfort; **Integrated Processes:** Nursing Process Assessment; **Client Need:** Physiological Integrity/Basic Care and Comfort/Assistive Devices; **Cognitive Level:** Application; **Reference:** Ignatavicius, D., & Workman, M. (2010), p. 1079.

47. ANSWER: 5, 2, 1, 6, 3, 4.

Containing the copious amounts of purulent drainage requires immediate attention for prevention of transmission of infectious organisms. Premedicating the client with pain medication before proceeding to other steps in the process allows time for the medication to be absorbed. Gathering all necessary supplies to change the dressing covering the wound allows unnecessary exposure of the open wound and sterile fields. Removing the soiled dressings and placing them in a closed bag for disposal prevents transmission of infectious organisms. Changing gloves after removing the soiled dressing, performing hand hygiene, and gloving before placing a sterile dressing, prevent contamination of the sterile dressings being applied.

TEST-TAKING TIP: Visualize the steps of the procedure prior to placing them in the correct order.

Content Area: Fundamentals; **Category of Health Alteration:** Basic Care and Comfort; **Integrated Processes**: Nursing Process Implementation; **Client Need:** Physiological Integrity/Basic Care and Comfort/Mobility/Immobility; **Cognitive Level:** Application; **Reference:** Black, J., & Hawks, J. (2009), p. 2050.

48. A nurse is evaluating a client's ability to perform active range of motion. Which illustration demonstrates the client's ability to correctly perform eversion?

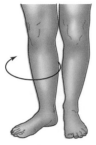

1.

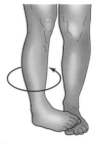

2.

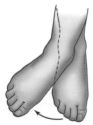

3.

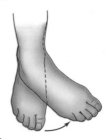

4.

49. A nurse is weighing the soiled diapers to determine the amount of fluid loss by an infant with diarrhea. The nurse subtracts a dry diaper weight of 0.2 grams from the weight of each soiled diaper. At the end of an 8-hour shift, the infant has had 5 soiled diapers weighing 6 grams and 5 soiled diapers weighing 5 grams. How many milliliters (mL) of fluid loss should the nurse have documented during the 8-hour shift?

_____ mL (Record your answer as a whole number.)

48. ANSWER: 3.

Illustration 3 shows eversion, which refers to turning outward. Illustration 1 shows external rotation; 2 is internal rotation; 4 is inversion, turning inward.

TEST-TAKING TIP: Use the memory cue that "inversion" is "in." Thus, "eversion" is "out." Eliminate options showing inversion and rotation.

Content Area: Fundamentals; **Category of Health Alteration:** Basic Care and Comfort; **Integrated Processes:** Nursing Process Evaluation; **Client Need:** Physiological Integrity/Basic Care and Comfort/Mobility/Immobility; **Cognitive Level:** Application; **Reference:** Potter, P., & Perry, A. (2009), pp. 1235–1236.

49. ANSWER: 53

Use a weight calculation to determine the amount of fluid loss. One gram of dry weight is equal to 1 mL of fluid loss. First, determine the weight of each soiled diaper (5 × 6 = 30 gram; 5 × 5 = 25 grams) and add these amounts together to get the total weight of the soiled diapers (30 + 25 = 55 grams). Then, multiply the weight of each dry diaper by the number of diapers soiled (10 × 0.2 = 2 grams) and subtract the total weight of the dry diapers from the total weight of the soiled diapers (55 − 2 = 53 grams). Finally, use the equivalency to determine that 53 grams is equivalent to 53 mL of fluid loss.

TEST-TAKING TIP: Use the formula 1 gram of dry weight = 1 mL of fluid. Do not forget to subtract the weight of each dry diaper.

Content Area: Fundamentals; **Category of Health Alteration:** Basic Care and Comfort; **Integrated Processes:** Communication and Documentation; **Client Need:** Physiological Integrity/Basic Care and Comfort/Elimination; **Cognitive Level:** Application; **Reference:** Ward, S., & Hisley, S. (2009), p. 688.

50. A client on low-flow oxygen therapy (2 liters per nasal cannula) is experiencing periods of difficulty breathing due to late-stage emphysema. Which interventions should a nurse plan to promote the client's oxygenation? **Select all that apply.**

1. Ensure a low level of noise in the environment.
2. Elevate the head of bed to 90 degrees.
3. Provide an overhead trapeze to change positions.
4. Position a tray table over the bed for the client to lean on that is cushioned with a pillow.
5. Provide frequent back and feet massages.
6. Increase the oxygen flow to 8 liters per minute.

51. A nurse is conversing with an 81-year-old client. Which statement reflects the nurse using an open-ended communication technique?

1. "You've said you have been coming to the clinic for a long time. When was your last visit to the clinic?"
2. "You are on a number of medications. Tell me how you keep track of what medication to take and when."
3. "You told me that you have increasing difficulty cooking and getting around the house. Would you like to start receiving meals in your home through Meals on Wheels?"
4. "I understand that you like to spend time outdoors. It will be important for you to wear sunscreen with a sun protection factor (SPF) of 15 or higher."

50. ANSWER: 2, 4.

The head of the bed elevated to 90 degrees and an over-the-bed tray table with a pillow for the client to lean on promotes lung expansion. A low level of noise in the environment may be helpful to the client with visual and ear difficulties. An overhead trapeze is used with orthopedic clients to change positions. A back or foot massage relaxes muscles in many diseases but has not been shown to improve breathing. Increasing the oxygen flow can decrease the client's drive to breathe.

TEST-TAKING TIP: Focus on the key words "promote oxygenation" and concentrate on the effect of each intervention. Eliminate options that do not promote oxygenation.

Content Area: Fundamentals; **Category of Health Alteration:** Basic Care and Comfort; **Integrated Processes:** Nursing Process Planning; **Client Need:** Physiological Integrity/Physiological Adaptation/Illness Management; **Cognitive Level:** Analysis; **Reference:** Black, J. & Hawks, J. (2009), p. 1582.

51. ANSWER: 2.

An open-ended therapeutic communication technique uses a broad question or statement that invites the client to elaborate. Option 1 is seeking additional information through clarifying time. Option 3 uses a closed-ended question that invites only a yes or no response. Option 4 is giving information.

TEST-TAKING TIP: An open-ended communication technique usually does not end with a question; thus eliminate options 1 and 3. Then eliminate option 4, which provides information.

Content Area: Fundamentals; **Category of Health Alteration:** Basic Care and Comfort; **Integrated Processes:** Caring; Communication and Documentation; **Client Need:** Psychosocial Integrity/Therapeutic Communications; **Cognitive Level:** Application; **References:** Berman, A., Snyder, S., Kozier, B., & Erb, G. (2008), pp. 469–471. Mauk, K. (2010). p. 114.

52. A nurse evaluates that a nursing assistant (NA) is able to correctly perform denture care for a client. In which order should the NA have demonstrated the denture care? Place each step in the correct numerical order (1–7).

_____ 1. Pushes the top denture up against the roof of the client's mouth.

_____ 2. Dons gloves and removes the client's dentures using a gauze pad.

_____ 3. Inspects the dentures for rough, worn, or sharp edges.

_____ 4. Moistens the top denture and inserts it at a slight tilt into the client's mouth.

_____ 5. Moistens the bottom denture, inserts, and then rotates it to fit the client's gum line.

_____ 6. Places a towel in the sink and cleanses the dentures under cool running water.

_____ 7. Inspects the client's mouth before insertion.

53. A parent calls a clinic about a child weighing 9.6 kg who has a temperature of 102.2°F (39°C) after receiving immunizations. The clinic protocol is to administer acetaminophen (Tylenol) 15 mg/kg every 4 to 6 hours as needed for fever. The parent has acetaminophen 160 mg/5 mL. How many milliliters (mL) should the nurse instruct the parent to administer for each dose?

_____ mL (Record your answer rounded to tenths.)

52. ANSWER: 2, 6, 3, 7, 4, 1, 5.
First the NA should don gloves and remove the client's dentures using a gauze pad. Then a towel should be placed in the sink and the denture cleansed under cool running water. During cleaning, the NA should inspect the dentures for rough, worn, or sharp edges. Before inserting the dentures, the NA should inspect the client's mouth for redness, irritation, lesions, or infections. Next, if the top denture is dry, the NA should moisten it and insert it at a slight tilt into the client's mouth. The NA should then push the top denture up against the roof of the client's mouth. Finally, the NA should moisten the bottom denture, insert, and then rotate it to fit the client's gum line. The bottom denture is inserted last because it is smaller. The NA should also ask if the dentures are comfortable.

TEST-TAKING TIP: Visualize providing denture care before placing the items in the correct order. Remember the bottom denture is inserted last.

Content Area: Fundamentals; **Category of Health Alteration:** Basic Care and Comfort; **Integrated Processes:** Nursing Process Evaluation; **Client Need:** Physiological Integrity/Basic Care and Comfort/Personal Hygiene; **Cognitive Level:** Application; **Reference:** Potter, P., & Perry, A. (2009), pp. 890–891.

53. ANSWER: 4.5
First determine the amount in milligrams for the child's weight:

15 mg: 1 kg :: X mg: 9.6 kg

X = 144 mg

Then determine the dose:

165 mg : 5 mL :: 144 mg : X mL

160X = 144 × 5

X = 720/160

X = 4.5 mL

TEST-TAKING TIP: Be sure to use the calculator provided on the exam and double-check your answer especially if it seems unusually large.

Content Area: Fundamentals; **Category of Health Alteration:** Medication Administration; **Integrated Processes:** Nursing Process Implementation; **Client Need:** Physiological Integrity/Pharmacological and Parenteral Therapies/Dosage Calculation; **Cognitive Level:** Analysis; **References:** Pickar, G., & Abernethy, A. (2008), p. 46; Berman, A., Snyder, S., & McKinney, D. (2011), pp. 652–659.

Test 6: Fundamentals: Medication Administration

54. Twelve hours after a client receives an initial dose of an antibiotic, a nurse enters the client's room to administer a second dose of the antibiotic by intravenous piggyback (IVPB). Place an X on the illustration where the nurse should attach the IVPB medication for administration.

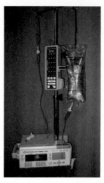

55. A health care provider orders furosemide (Lasix) 30 mg IV now. The medication is supplied in a 40 mg per 2-mL vial. How much medication should the nurse withdraw into a 3-mL syringe? Place an X on the appropriate location on the syringe.

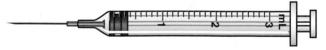

54. ANSWER: X.

In IVPB administration, a secondary line is used for medication administration. The tubing is attached to the primary solution's tubing in the upper port above the pump. Lowering the primary solution ensures that the IVPB medication will be administered by gravity flow first, and then the primary infusion will resume.

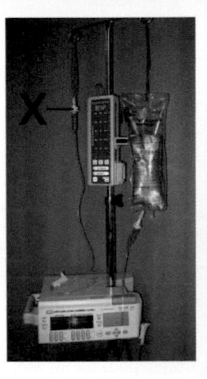

TEST-TAKING TIP: Focus on the illustration and the directions in the item stem to select the correct site for attaching the IVPB to the tubing for administration.

Content Area: Fundamentals; **Category of Health Alteration:** Medication Administration; **Integrated Processes:** Nursing Process Implementation; **Client Need:** Physiological Integrity/Pharmacological and Parenteral Therapies/Medication Administration; **Cognitive Level:** Application; **Reference:** Berman, A., Snyder, S., & McKinney, D. (2011), p. 693.

55. ANSWER:

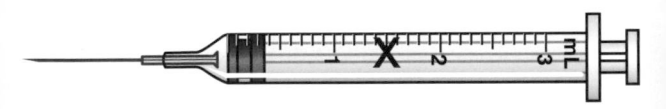

$$\frac{30 \text{ mg}}{40 \text{ mg}} \times 2 \text{ mL} = 1.5 \text{ mL}$$

TEST-TAKING TIP: Read the question carefully to properly set up the formula. [(Dose ordered ÷ dose on hand) × amount on hand = amount to administer] Then locate the 1.5 mL on the syringe.

Content Area: Fundamentals; **Category of Health Alteration:** Medication Administration; **Integrated Processes:** Nursing Process Implementation; **Client Need:** Physiological Integrity/Pharmacological and Parenteral Therapies/Dosage Calculation; **Cognitive Level:** Application; **Reference:** Potter, P., & Perry, A. (2009), pp. 697, 735.

56. A client has multiple medications prescribed by a health care provider (HCP). Which prescriptions should a nurse clarify with the HCP? **Select all that apply.**

1. Heparin 5,000 IU SC bid
2. Lisinopril (Prinivil) .5 mg oral daily
3. Hydrochlorothiazide (Microzide) 12.5 mg oral daily
4. MS 2–4 mg IV q1h prn for pain
5. Levothyroxine (Levoxyl) 100 mcg oral daily

57. A nurse assesses that a client's dyspnea, fatigue, and skin color have improved after receiving two units of packed red blood cells (PRBCs). Which serum laboratory values should the nurse review to also evaluate the effectiveness of the PRBCs? **Select all that apply.**

1. Platelet count
2. Serum albumin
3. White blood cell counts
4. Hemoglobin
5. Hematocrit

56. ANSWER: 1, 2, 4.
Prescriptions that use abbreviations included on The Joint Commission's list of dangerous abbreviations, acronyms, and symbols must be clarified with the HCP. The abbreviation IU, intended to mean international unit, can be mistaken as IV (intravenous), and "units" should be used. A dose of medication with an absent 0 can be mistaken for 5 mg, and a 0 before a decimal point should be used when the dose is less than 1. The abbreviation MS can be mistaken for morphine sulfate or magnesium sulfate. The complete medication name should be used in the order. The orders for hydrochlorothiazide and levothyroxine use the complete drug name and have the correct dose, abbreviations, route, and frequency.

TEST-TAKING TIP: Look for options that contain items included on The Joint Commission's "Do Not Use" list of abbreviations, acronyms, and symbols.

Content Area: Fundamentals; **Category of Health Alteration:** Medication Administration; **Integrated Processes:** Nursing Process Implementation; **Client Need:** Physiological Integrity/Pharmacological and Parenteral Therapies/ Medication Administration; **Cognitive Level:** Analysis; **Reference:** Potter, P., & Perry, A. (2009), pp. 701–703; **EBP Reference:** Institute for Safe Medication Practices (ISMP). (2010). *ISMP's List of Error-Prone Abbreviations, Symbols, and Dose Designations*. Retrieved from www.ismp.org/Tools/errorproneabbreviations.pdf

57. ANSWER: 4, 5.
Hemoglobin and hematocrit measure the effect of administering packed red blood cells. One unit of packed red blood cells will raise the hemoglobin level 1 gram. Platelet count is used to evaluate the effect of platelet administration. Serum albumin is used to evaluate nutritional status or fluid shifts from intracellular to extracellular compartments. White blood cell counts are used to evaluate the presence of an infection. Red blood cell count is used to evaluate the effectiveness of administering PRBCs.

TEST-TAKING TIP: Focus on what each test measures and eliminate options that do not pertain to blood cells. Then eliminate the laboratory finding that is used to evaluate the presence of an infection.

Content Area: Fundamentals; **Category of Health Alteration:** Medication Administration; **Integrated Processes:** Nursing Process Evaluation; **Client Need:** Physiological Integrity/Pharmacological and Parenteral Therapies/Blood and Blood Products; **Cognitive Level:** Application; **Reference:** Black, J., & Hawks, J. (2009), p. 2005.

58. A client is to receive albuterol (Proventil) 2 puffs qid with a spacer. Place an X on the item the nurse should plan to retrieve to correctly administer the medication to the client.

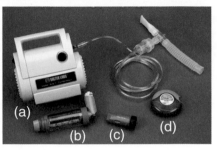

59. A nurse is preparing 100 mg methylprednisolone sodium succinate (Solu-Medrol) in preparation for a client's chemotherapy treatment. The medication is supplied in a 125 mg per 2 mL Mix-O-Vial®. How many milliliters (mL) should the nurse prepare to administer?

_____ mL (Record your answer rounded to tenths.)

58. ANSWER:

A spacer (aerochamber) traps medication released from the inhaler, and then the client inhales the medication from the device. The spacer breaks up and slows down the medication particles, enhancing the amount of medication received by the client. Device "a" is a handheld ultrasonic nebulizer that mixes

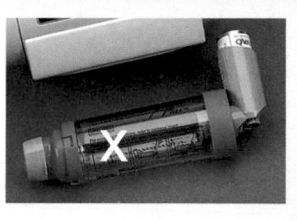

a small volume of medication with normal saline. The device forces air through the nebulizer to deliver the medication and humidity as a fine mist for deep lung inhalation. Device "c" is a dry powder inhaler, and device "d" is a diskhaler.

TEST-TAKING TIP: If unsure, eliminate options that would not have an extra device between the medication to be delivered and the client's mouth. Of the two remaining options, eliminate the device that would humidify the medication.

Content Area: Fundamentals; **Category of Health Alteration:** Medication Administration; **Integrated Processes:** Nursing Process Planning; **Client Need:** Safe and Effective Care Environment/Safety and Infection Control/Safe Use of Equipment; **Cognitive Level:** Application; **Reference:** Potter, P., & Perry, A. (2009), p. 733.

59. ANSWER: 1.6

Use a proportion formula:

125 mg : 2 mL :: 100 mg : X mL

Multiply the extremes (outside values) and means (inside values) and solve for X.

125 X = 200

X = 1.6 mL

TEST-TAKING TIP: Read the question carefully to properly set up the formula. If the amount seems unusually large, recheck your calculations.

Content Area: Fundamentals; **Category of Health Alteration:** Medication Administration; **Integrated Processes:** Nursing Process Implementation; **Client Need:** Physiological Integrity/Pharmacological and Parenteral Therapies/ Dosage Calculation; **Cognitive Level:** Application; **Reference:** Pickar, G., & Abernethy, A. (2008), p. 46.

60. After correctly completing the five rights of medication administration, performing hand hygiene, and positioning the client, which steps should a nurse take to administer a subcutaneous injection to an average-sized client? Place each step in the correct numerical order (1–7).

_____ 1. Dispose the syringe in a sharps container.

_____ 2. Apply gloves and locate the injection site using anatomical landmarks.

_____ 3. Remove the needle cap by pulling it straight off.

_____ 4. Inject the needle quickly and inject the medication slowly.

_____ 5. Hold the syringe as a dart and pinch the skin with the nondominant hand.

_____ 6. Reposition the client in a comfortable position.

_____ 7. Cleanse the site using an antiseptic swab.

61. A nurse is teaching a parent to administer an acetaminophen (Tylenol) suppository to a 6-month-old infant who is febrile. Which statements should be included in the nurse's instructions? **Select all that apply.**

1. "Apply a glove and lubricate the suppository if it is not already lubricated."

2. "Insert the suppository gently with your little finger to the depth of your first knuckle."

3. "Tightly clamp your infant's buttocks together after administration."

4. "Observe that the suppository results in a bowel movement."

5. "Ensure that the suppository is past the infant's anal sphincter and against the intestinal wall."

60. ANSWER: 2, 7, 3, 5, 4, 1, 6.
First, apply gloves and locate the injection site using anatomical land-marks. Then cleanse the site using an antiseptic swab. Start at the center of the site and rotate outward in a circular direction. Remove the needle cap by pulling it straight off. Next, hold the syringe as a dart and pinch the skin with the nondominant hand. Inject the needle quickly and inject the medication slowly. Finally, dispose the syringe in a sharps container and reposition the client in a comfortable position.

TEST-TAKING TIP: Visualize the procedure before attempting to place the steps in the correct order.

Content Area: Fundamentals; **Category of Health Alteration:** Medication Administration; **Integrated Processes:** Nursing Process Implementation; **Client Need:** Physiological Integrity/Pharmacological and Parenteral Therapies/ Medication Administration; **Cognitive Level:** Application; **Reference:** Potter, P., & Perry, A. (2009), pp. 746–747.

61. ANSWER: 1, 2, 5.
The parent should apply a glove and lubricate the suppository with a water-soluble lubricating jelly if it is not already lubricated. The parent should insert the suppository gently, but quickly, approximately as far as the first knuckle of the little finger and beyond the anal sphincter. The finger should then be withdrawn and the infant's buttocks held together gently (not tightly) until the infant's urge to evacuate the suppository passes. The purpose of acetaminophen is to lower the infant's temperature and not induce defecation.

TEST-TAKING TIP: First, visualize the steps prior to identifying the options to address with the parent. Consider the action of acetaminophen to eliminate an option.

Content Area: Fundamentals; **Category of Health Alteration:** Medication Administration; **Integrated Processes:** Teaching and Learning; **Client Need:** Physiological Integrity/Pharmacological and Parenteral Therapies/Medication Administration; **Cognitive Level:** Application; **Reference:** Potter, P., & Perry, A. (2009), p. 731.

62. A client weighing 132 pounds is to receive a loading dose of phenytoin (Dilantin) intravenously. The client is to receive 20 mg/kg in three divided doses in 2-hour intervals. In order to give the correct dose, how many milligrams (mg) should the nurse administer at each dose?

_____ mg (Record your answer as a whole number.)

63. A new nurse is administering medications to various clients. In which situations should an experienced nurse intervene? **Select all that apply.**

1. Takes a client's blood pressure, dons gloves, and then administers a sublingual nitroglycerin tablet under the tongue of a client experiencing chest pain.
2. Writes a telephone order as a health care provider (HCP) states it, thanks the HCP for the order, and then immediately implements the order as written.
3. Shakes a container of liquid medication, pours the dose while holding the medication cup, then rests the cup on a flat surface to measure the dose at eye level.
4. Crushes an enteric-coated aspirin tablet and mixes it with applesauce to administer to a client experiencing dysphagia.
5. Uses a pill cutter and cuts a scored tablet in half to administer metoprolol (Lopressor) 12.5 mg oral when the available dose is 50 mg.

62. ANSWER: 400

Convert pounds to kilograms. One kilogram equals 2.2 pounds (132 ÷ 2.2 = 60 kg). Then determine total dose (20 mg × 60 kg = 1200 mg). Then determine amount for each dose (1200 mg ÷ 3 = 400 mg).

TEST-TAKING TIP: Identify what the question is asking (administering one dose of medication) and the key components (client's weight, amount of medication ordered, and number of doses). Identifying these elements and applying dosage calculations are necessary to answer this question.

Content Area: Fundamentals; **Category of Health Alteration:** Medication Administration; **Integrated Processes:** Nursing Process Analysis; **Client Need:** Physiological Integrity/Pharmacological and Parenteral Therapies/Dosage Calculation; **Cognitive Level:** Analysis; **Reference:** Berman, A., Snyder, S., & McKinney, D. (2011), p. 661.

63. ANSWER: 2, 4, 5.

The nurse should write the complete telephone order as delivered, read it back to the HCP, and receive confirmation of its accuracy from the HCP. An enteric-coated medication should not be crushed. The nurse should cut the scored metoprolol tablet into fourths and give one-fourth of a tablet or obtain a smaller dose from pharmacy. The blood pressure should be determined prior to administering nitroglycerin sublingually (under the tongue) because it can cause hypotension. Shaking ensures that the medication is mixed and placing the medication cup on a flat surface and reading the dose at eye level ensures that the meniscus of the liquid medication is level with and read at the appropriate line on the cup.

TEST-TAKING TIP: The key word is "intervene." Select the options with incorrectly performed actions.

Content Area: Fundamentals; **Category of Health Alteration:** Medication Administration; **Integrated Processes:** Nursing Process Evaluation; **Client Need:** Physiological Integrity/Pharmacological and Parenteral Therapies/Medication Administration; **Cognitive Level:** Analysis; **Reference:** Potter, P., & Perry, A. (2009), pp. 694, 699, 720–722.

64. A nurse is documenting the administration of an intramuscular (IM) medication into the site illustrated. Which site should the nurse document for the IM injection?

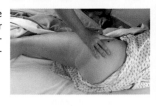

1. Left vastis lateralis muscle
2. Left dorsogluteal muscle
3. Left ventrogluteal muscle
4. Left rectus femoris muscle

65. A nurse is to administer two oral medication tablets through a percutaneous endoscopic gastrostomy (PEG) tube to a client also receiving continuous enteral feeding. Which steps should be taken by the nurse when safely administering tablets through a PEG tube? Place each step in the correct numerical order (1–7).

_____ 1. Crush the first tablet and mix it in 20 mL of water.
_____ 2. Flush the PEG tube with 30 mL of water.
_____ 3. Administer the medication.
_____ 4. Verify that the medication can be crushed and given through an enteral tube.
_____ 5. Follow medication administration by flushing the tube with 30 mL of water and resume feeding.
_____ 6. Place the continuous feeding pump on hold.
_____ 7. Check for residual volume.

64. ANSWER: 3.

The left ventrogluteal site is located in the lateral hip in the middle of a triangle formed by placing the right palm on the greater trochanter, the index finger on the anterior superior iliac spine, and the middle finger spread wide and pointing toward the iliac crest. The left vastis lateralis injection site is located in the middle third of the anterolateral thigh. The left dorsogluteal injection site is located in the right upper outer quadrant of the buttocks, above an imaginary line from the posterior superior iliac spine to the greater trochanter and 2 to 3 inches below the iliac crest. The left rectus femoris muscle is located in the middle third of the anterior thigh; it should not be used unless no other medication routes are feasible.

TEST-TAKING TIP: If unsure, identify the preferred injection site for an intramuscular injection.

Content Area: Fundamentals; **Category of Health Alteration:** Medication Administration; **Integrated Processes:** Communication and Documentation; **Client Need:** Physiological Integrity/Pharmacological and Parenteral Therapies/ Medication Administration; **Cognitive Level:** Application; **Reference:** Potter, P., & Perry, A. (2009), pp. 751–752.

65. ANSWER: 4, 1, 6, 7, 2, 3, 5.

Before giving medications via enteral tubes, the nurse should always determine if a medication can be crushed and administered via an enteral feeding tube. Once the medication is crushed, it should be mixed with 20 mL to 30 mL of water to allow it to dissolve. Place the feeding pump on hold. Before administration of anything into an enteral tube, residual volume should be assessed. The PEG should be flushed before and after the medication administration to remove formula residue which may interact with the medication and cause blockage of the tube. This also assures tube patency.

TEST-TAKING TIP: Visualize the steps in giving medications through a PEG tube. Prioritizing is placing items in the correct sequence.

Content Area: Fundamentals; **Category of Health Alteration:** Medication Administration; **Integrated Processes:** Nursing Process Implementation; **Client Need:** Physiological Integrity/Pharmacological and Parenteral Therapies/ Medication Administration; **Cognitive Level:** Analysis; **Reference:** Smeltzer, S., Bare, B., Hinkle, J., & Cheever, K. (2010), pp. 1027–1029.

66. A 50-year-old client has an order to receive prochlorperazine (Compazine) 10 mg IM now. Which steps should a nurse include when withdrawing the medication from the ampule? **Select all that apply.**

1. Tap the ampule top to move fluid from the neck of the ampule into the ampule.
2. Place a gauze pad above the neck of the ampule and snap the neck away from the hands.
3. Apply a filter needle to a syringe to withdraw the medication.
4. Inject air into the ampule to withdraw the medication.
5. Hold the ampule upside down and insert the needle into the center of the ampule opening.
6. Remove the filter needle from the syringe, replacing it with a 1½ inch needle.

67. A nurse is monitoring a client receiving total parenteral nutrition (TPN). Which findings should prompt the nurse to notify the health care provider that the client is experiencing adverse effects from the TPN? **Select all that apply.**

1. White blood cell count 13,000/mm³
2. Blood glucose 180 mg/dL
3. Urine output 5600 mL past 24 hours
4. Abdomen distended
5. Mucous membranes dry
6. Gastric emptying delayed

66. ANSWER: 1, 2, 3, 5, 6.
A light and quick tap of the top will move fluid into the ampule. If fluid remains in the top and neck, there may be an inadequate amount. Use of a gauze pad and snapping the ampule neck away from the hands protects the nurse's fingers and face if the glass were to shatter. A filter needle is required to prevent aspiration of glass fragments. Fluid can be aspirated from an inverted ampule, but touching the rim contaminates the needle and can result in solution dripping out alongside the needle. The filter needle should be removed before administration to prevent possible glass particles from being administered. A 1½ inch needle is the correct length for an intramuscular (IM) injection. Injecting air into the ampule forces fluid out of the ampule and medication will be lost.

TEST-TAKING TIP: Visualize the steps prior to reading the options. Eliminate the one step that would pertain to a vial and not an ampule.

Content Area: Fundamentals; **Category of Health Alteration:** Medication Administration; **Integrated Processes:** Nursing Process Implementation; **Client Need:** Physiological Integrity/Pharmacological and Parenteral Therapies/ Medication Administration; **Cognitive Level:** Application; **Reference:** Potter, P., & Perry, A. (2009), pp. 738–739.

67. ANSWER: 1, 2, 3, 5.
An elevated WBC suggests an infection. A high glucose concentration of the TPN solution makes it an ideal culture medium for bacterial and fungal growth. TPN solutions are 10% to 50% dextrose in water. High glucose content in the TPN solution can lead to hyperglycemia. Hyperglycemia can cause diuresis, excessive fluid loss, and dehydration. Excess glucose is excreted by the renal tubules, pulling large volumes of water into the tubules via osmosis, resulting in a large volume of urine output (hyperosmolar diuresis). Abdominal distention and delayed gastric emptying are adverse effects associated with enteral feedings and not TPN.

TEST-TAKING TIP: Eliminate options that are associated with enteral and not parenteral nutrition. Recall that TPN has a high glucose content.

Content Area: Adult Health; **Category of Health Alteration:** Nutrition; **Integrated Processes:** Nursing Process Evaluation; **Client Need:** Physiological Integrity/Pharmacological and Parenteral Therapies/Total Parenteral Nutrition; **Cognitive Level:** Application; **References:** Berman, A., Snyder, S., Kozier, B., & Erb, G. (2008), p. 1277; Smeltzer, S., Bare, B., Hinkle, J., & Cheever, K. (2010), pp. 1034–1037.

68. An adult client visits a clinic to receive a hepatitis B vaccine. Which anatomical location **recommended** by the Centers for Disease Control and Prevention (CDC) should the nurse assess and select for administering the injection?

Ventrogluteal site

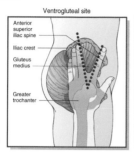

1.

Deltoid site

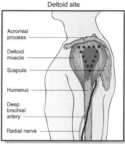

2.

Vastus lateralis site

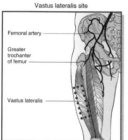

3.

Dorsogluteal site

4.

68. ANSWER: 2.

The deltoid muscle is on the lateral aspect of the upper arm and is a recommended site for hepatitis B vaccination in adults. Studies have shown a suboptimal response when administered in the gluteal muscle sites. The anterolateral thigh is recommended for infants and neonates. Option 1 is the ventrogluteal site. Option 3 is the vastis lateralis muscle. Option 4 is the dorsogluteal site.

TEST-TAKING TIP: Focus on the key words "recommended" and "hepatitis B vaccine." Think about the location of most vaccines for adults.

Content Area: Fundamentals; **Category of Health Alteration:** Medication Administration; **Integrated Processes:** Nursing Process Assessment; **Client Need:** Health Promotion and Maintenance/Health and Wellness; Physiological Integrity/Pharmacological and Parenteral Therapies/Medication Administration; **Cognitive Level:** Application; **Reference:** Berman, A., Snyder, S., & McKinney, D. (2011), pp. 685–688; **EBP Reference:** Centers for Disease Control and Prevention. (2009). *Epidemiology and Prevention of Vaccine-Preventable Diseases*. Atkinson, W., Wolfe, S., Hamborsky, J., & McIntyre, L. (Eds., 11th ed.). Washington, DC: Public Health Foundation. Retrieved from www.cdc.gov/vaccines/pubs/pinkbook/downloads/hepb.pdf.

Test 7: Fundamentals: Safety, Disaster Preparedness, and Infection Control

69. A nurse is using a motorized lift to assist a client from a chair to the toilet. Place an X on the illustration where the lift is being used improperly.

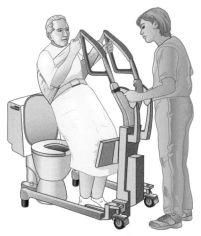

70. A nurse is preparing to administer diazepam (Valium) 10 mg IV to a client experiencing status epilepticus. The medication is supplied in a vial labeled 20 mg/2 mL. How many milliliters (mL) should the nurse prepare for administration?

_____ mL (Record your answer as a whole number.)

69. ANSWER:
The client should be grasping the handles and not the safety straps. Grasping the safety straps can result in client injury.

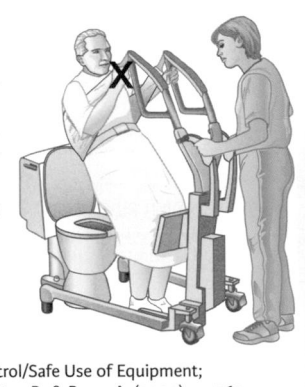

TEST-TAKING TIP: Examine the picture carefully. The client, rather than the nurse, is performing an unsafe action for which the nurse should be observing.

Content Area: Fundamentals; **Category of Health Alteration:** Safety, Disaster Preparedness, and Infection Control; **Integrated Processes:** Nursing Process Evaluation; **Client Need:** Safe and Effective Care Environment/Safety and Infection Control/Safe Use of Equipment; **Cognitive Level:** Application; **Reference:** Potter, P., & Perry, A. (2009), p. 1263.

70. ANSWER: 1
Use a proportion formula:

20 mg : 2 mL :: 10 mg : X mL

Multiply the extremes (outside values) and the means (inside values) and solve for X.

20 X = 20

X = 1 mL

TEST-TAKING TIP: Use a proportion formula and solve for X. If the amount seems unusually large, recheck your calculations. You should be able to recognize that 10 is $\frac{1}{2}$ of 20.

Content Area: Fundamentals; **Category of Health Alteration:** Safety, Disaster Preparedness, and Infection Control; **Integrated Processes:** Nursing Process Implementation; **Client Need:** Physiological Integrity/Pharmacological and Parenteral Therapies/Dosage Calculation; **Cognitive Level:** Analysis; **Reference:** Pickar, G., & Abernethy, A. (2008), p. 46.

71. A student nurse is taking the blood pressure of a 3-year-old child. Which actions indicate that the student nurse needs additional teaching to take an accurate blood pressure (BP) reading? **Select all that apply.**

1. The inflatable bladder length covers 50% of the circumference of the child's arm.
2. The child sits in his or her mother's lap while the BP is taken.
3. The child's BP is taken immediately after entering the exam room.
4. The child is sitting on the exam table during a second BP reading and his or her legs are uncrossed.
5. The BP is taken while the child's arm is located at heart level.
6. The stethoscope is placed gently on the antecubital fossa.

72. A nurse is completing a fall assessment scale on a 72-year-old client who is currently confused and has impaired judgment. The client usually wears glasses and a hearing aid, but both were forgotten at home. The client has no history of falling. The client takes furosemide (Lasix) for blood pressure control and experiences urgency and postural hypotension with dizziness when getting up too fast. Based on the Fall Assessment Tool, which score should the nurse assign to the client?

Client Factor	Score
History of falls	15
Confusion	5
Age over 65	5
Impaired judgment	5
Sensory deficit	5
Decreased level of consciousness	5
Increased anxiety	5
Incontinence/urgency	5
Medications affecting blood pressure	5
Postural hypotension with dizziness	5
Environmental factors: Attached equipment	5

71. ANSWER: 1, 3.
The inflatable bladder length should cover 80–100% of the circumference of the child's arm. A too large cuff size results in a lower BP reading. Before the BP measurement is taken there should be at least 5 minutes of rest in a sitting position. The child should be in a sitting position; in the mother's lap is acceptable. A sitting position is correct and legs should be uncrossed. The child's arm should be level with his or her heart. Raising or lowering the arm can result in a too low or a too high reading. A stethoscope that is placed too firmly on the antecubital fossa causes errors in auscultation.

TEST-TAKING TIP: When selecting options, consider that a cuff that is too large will result in a lower BP and that activity immediately prior to a BP measurement will result in a higher BP.

Content Area: Fundamentals; **Category of Health Alteration:** Safety, Disaster Preparedness, and Infection Control; **Integrated Processes:** Nursing Process Evaluation; **Client Need:** Safe and Effective Care Environment/Safety and Infection Control/Safe Use of Equipment; **Cognitive Level:** Application; **Reference:** Potter, P., & Perry, A. (2009), pp. 539–545; **EBP Reference:** Cincinnati Children's Hospital Medical Center. (2009). *Best evidence statement (BESt). Blood pressure measurement in children.* Retrieved from www.guideline.gov/summary/summary.aspx?ss=15&doc_id =14293&nbr=7169.

72. ANSWER: 35
Confusion (5), age (5), impaired judgment (5), sensory deficit (5), urgency (5), blood pressure medications (5), and postural hypotension (5).

TEST-TAKING TIP: When reading the situation, be sure to consider that both hearing and sight are scored together with one score for sensory deficit.

Content Area: Fundamentals; **Category of Health Alteration:** Safety, Disaster Preparedness, and Infection Control; **Integrated Processes:** Nursing Process Assessment; **Client Need:** Safe and Effective Care Environment/Safety and Infection Control/Accident and Injury Prevention; **Cognitive Level:** Application; **Reference:** Potter, P., & Perry, A. (2009), p. 820.

73. A client who is confused and agitated persistently attempts to get out of bed despite using least restrictive methods to protect the client. A health care provider (HCP) prescribes a restraint to protect the client from falling out of bed. In this situation, which type of restraint is **best** for the nurse to apply?

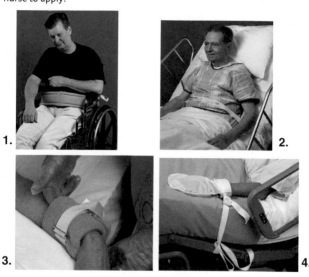

1.

2.

3.

4.

73. ANSWER: 2.

A vest restraint is used mainly to prevent a client from getting out of bed unassisted or from falling out of a wheelchair. It is best because it allows free movement of the hands and arms but restricts movement of the torso. A belt restraint (Illustration 1) is used to prevent a client from falling when getting up from a chair or wheelchair and helps to remind the client not to get up unassisted. Because it is smaller, it provides less protection. Wrist (Illustration 3) or mitt restraints (Illustration 4) are used mainly to prevent a client from pulling at tubes such as IV lines or nasogastric tubes. Although these may prevent a client from getting out of bed, they can increase client agitation.

TEST-TAKING TIP: Select an option that is the least restrictive type of restraint that would protect the client from falling out of bed.

Content Area: Fundamentals; **Category of Health Alteration:** Safety, Disaster Preparedness, and Infection Control; **Integrated Processes:** Nursing Process Implementation; **Client Need:** Safe and Effective Care Environment/Safety and Infection Control/Use of Restraints/Safety Devices; **Cognitive Level:** Application; **Reference:** Potter, P., & Perry, A. (2009), pp. 834–839.

74. A nurse completes teaching with a client about home safety and guidelines for electrical shock prevention. Which statements made by the client indicate that further teaching is needed? **Select all that apply.**

1. "I should avoid running electrical wires under carpeting."
2. "I should attach extension cords together from one electrical outlet to reduce the number of cords that need to be secured to the floor."
3. "I should disconnect electrical cords before cleaning an item, such as my toaster."
4. "I should grasp the cord, not the plug, when unplugging electrical items."
5. "I should read the owner's manual before operating unfamiliar or new equipment or electrical items."

75. A new nursing assistant (NA) is delivering meal trays and begins to enter a client's room. The client's door has the sign illustrated posted outside the door. Which action should be taken by a nurse observing the nursing assistant's actions?

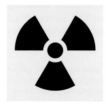

1. Obtain the tray from the NA, put on non-latex gloves, and deliver the meal tray.
2. Inform the NA that the NA's entry is prohibited because radioactive materials are present.
3. Inform the NA that a procedure is in progress and to wait to deliver the tray until the sign is removed.
4. Inform the NA that the client has an infectious disease and that a gown, gloves, and N-95 filter mask are required before entry.

74. ANSWER: 2, 4.
Extension cords should be used only when necessary. Multiple extension cords from one outlet increase the risk of overheating. The plug, and not the cord, should be grasped when unplugging electrical items. Running electrical wires under carpeting should be avoided. Electrical cords should be disconnected prior to cleaning an item. Reading the owner's manual prior to operating unfamiliar electrical equipment reduces the chance of an injury from improper use.

TEST-TAKING TIP: The key phrase is "needs further teaching." Select statements that are incorrect.

Content Area: Fundamentals; **Category of Health Alteration:** Safety, Disaster Preparedness, and Infection Control; **Integrated Processes:** Teaching and Learning; **Client Need:** Safe and Effective Care Environment/Safety and Infection Control/ Home Safety; **Cognitive Level:** Application; **Reference:** Potter, P., & Perry, A. (2009), p. 842.

75. ANSWER: 2.
The sign illustrated is a radiation warning symbol. Only personnel experienced in radiation therapy should be entering the client's room. Personnel should wear a dosimeter, which measures the amount of radiation exposure. Care should be rotated among experienced nurses to minimize exposure. Non-latex gloves are ineffective protection for radiation exposure. Gloves would be worn if this were an infectious hazard sign. The length of time that radiation material is left in place varies from a few hours to several days. Rather than waiting to deliver the meal tray, an experienced nurse should deliver it. The symbol for an infectious hazard is different in appearance from this sign.

TEST-TAKING TIP: If unsure of the answer, select the option that would best protect the nursing assistant's safety.

Content Area: Fundamentals; **Category of Health Alteration:** Safety, Disaster Preparedness, and Infection Control; **Integrated Processes:** Nursing Process Implementation; **Client Need:** Safe and Effective Care Environment/Safety and Infection Control/Handling Hazardous and Infectious Materials; **Cognitive Level:** Analysis; **Reference:** Osborn, S., Wraa, C., & Watson, A. (2010), p. 2086.

76. A client is at risk for falls related to left-sided weakness. Which nursing interventions should a nurse include when developing a plan of care for the client? **Select all that apply.**

1. Implement fall precautions such as activating the client's bed alarm.
2. Make hourly rounds to the client to determine needs.
3. Offer copious liquids throughout the day and evening shifts.
4. Assist the client to the toilet every 2 hours.
5. Stand on the client's right side when assisting with ambulation.

77. A nurse is using a board with graphic symbols when communicating with a male client who has receptive aphasia and neutropenia. Which illustration from a communication board would **best** assist the nurse when teaching the client about the priority action to prevent an infection?

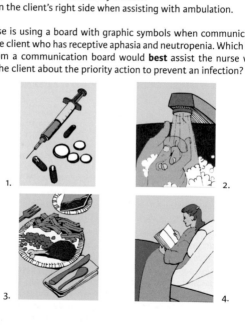

1.

2.

3.

4.

76. ANSWER: 1, 2, 4.

Fall precautions include using an alert system, such as a bed alarm, to notify health care personnel that the client is attempting to get out of bed. Hourly rounding provides a means to check on the client and address any needs prior to the client attempting to get out of bed independently and risking a fall. Toileting every 2 hours will help to reduce the chance that the client will attempt to get out of bed without assistance to use the bathroom. Liquids should be avoided during the late evening to reduce the need for night-time urination. Because the client is weak on the left side, health care personnel should stand on the client's weaker side to provide support and help prevent a fall.

TEST-TAKING TIP: Read each option carefully to determine whether it would increase or decrease the risk of a fall. Eliminate options that can increase the risk for a fall.

Content Area: Fundamentals; **Category of Health Alteration:** Safety, Disaster Preparedness, and Infection Control; **Integrated Processes:** Nursing Process Planning; **Client Need:** Safe and Effective Care Environment/Safety and Infection Control/Accident and Injury Prevention; **Cognitive Level:** Application; **Reference:** Potter, P., & Perry, A. (2009), pp. 823, 829. **EBP Reference:** Meade, C., Bursell, A., & Ketelsen, L. (2006). Effects of nursing rounds on patients' call light use, satisfaction and safety, *American Journal of Nursing*, 106(9), 58.

77. ANSWER: 2.

Clients can easily come in contact with microorganisms in the environment that can cause infection. Bacterial counts on the hands can be reduced by rigorous hand hygiene. Taking medications as prescribed, eating a healthy diet, and getting sufficient rest are other measures that help to prevent infection, but hand washing is the priority when a client has a low neutrophil count (neutropenia).

TEST-TAKING TIP: The key words are "best" and "priority action." Select the option that immediately reduces bacterial counts.

Content Area: Fundamentals; **Category of Health Alteration:** Safety, Disaster Preparedness, and Infection Control; **Integrated Processes:** Communication and Documentation; **Client Need:** Safe and Effective Care Environment/Safety and Infection Control/Standard Precautions/Transmission-Based Precautions/Surgical Asepsis; **Cognitive Level:** Application; **Reference:** Potter, P., & Perry, A. (2009), pp. 653–654.

78. A client with dementia from Alzheimer's disease is being cared for in the home by the client's spouse. A home health nurse is assessing the home environment. Which findings should the nurse recommend that the spouse **modify**? **Select all that apply.**

1. Throw rugs in front of doorways and sinks
2. Protective door handle covers on doors opening to the outside
3. Nonskid mat and a shower chair in the shower stall
4. Cleaning supplies and medicines stored in separate lockable cupboards
5. Graspable handrail that is smoothly shaped the same from top to bottom on all stairways

79. A nurse is assessing the function of a client's Pleur-evac chest drainage system. Place an X on the area the nurse should check when determining the presence of an air leak.

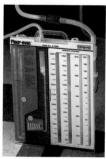

78. ANSWER: 1, 5.

Throw rugs should be removed because they can predispose to tripping and falls. The end of the handrail on stairs should be shaped differently to alert the person of the end of the stairs. Door handle covers will keep the person from wandering outdoors unattended. Nonskid mat and a chair will prevent falls when showering. Keeping chemicals and medicines locked and in different locations prevents accidental poisoning.

TEST-TAKING TIP: The key word is "modify." Read each option and select those that pose a safety risk to the client.

Content Area: Fundamentals; **Category of Health Alteration:** Safety, Disaster Preparedness, and Infection Control; **Integrated Processes:** Nursing Process Assessment; **Client Need:** Safe and Effective Care Environment/Safety and Infection Control/Accident and Injury Prevention; **Cognitive Level:** Analysis; **Reference:** Berman, A., Snyder, S., & McKinney, D. (2011), p. 579.

79. ANSWER:

The second chamber is the water-seal chamber. Continuous bubbling in this chamber is unexpected and indicates a leak between the client and the water seal. The air leak could be inside the client's thorax, at the chest tube insertion site, between tubing connections, or within the system. In the wet suction illustrated, constant, gentle bubbling should occur in the first chamber (the suction-control chamber) when using suction.

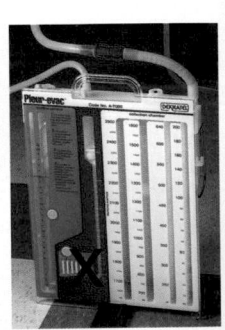

TEST-TAKING TIP: This is a wet suction; eliminate the chamber where bubbling is normally observed. Then eliminate the collection chamber where the collection tubing enters the chamber. The remaining chamber is the water-seal chamber.

Content Area: Fundamentals; **Category of Health Alteration:** Safety, Disaster Preparedness, and Infection Control; **Integrated Processes:** Nursing Process Assessment; **Client Need:** Physiological Integrity/Reduction of Risk Potential/Therapeutic Procedures; Safe and Effective Care Environment/Safety and Infection Control/Safe Use of Equipment; **Cognitive Level:** Application; **Reference:** Potter, P., & Perry, A. (2009), pp. 952–955.

80. A high-school student is brought to a school nurse's office after getting a chemical splashed in an eye during a biology lab. Which actions should the nurse take to treat the student? Place each action in the correct numerical order (1–6).

_____ 1. Arrange for transport to an emergency department.
_____ 2. While forcefully keeping the eye open, use clean cold water to gently rinse the eye.
_____ 3. Irrigate the eye copiously for 20 minutes, evert the upper lid to flush the eye thoroughly.
_____ 4. Discuss the situation with the student's parents.
_____ 5. Inform the student of the actions that must be taken.
_____ 6. Have the student lie on a flat surface.

81. A client is experiencing status epilepticus. Which actions should a nurse take when caring for this client? **Select all that apply.**

1. Close the curtains around the client's bed.
2. Restrain the client's head and arms.
3. Insert an oral airway when the client's jaw is relaxed.
4. Loosen the client's clothing.
5. Turn the client on his or her side with the head flexed slightly forward.
6. Remove all pillows and blankets from the client's bed.

80. ANSWER: 5, 6, 2, 3, 4, 1.
First, inform the student of the actions that must be taken. Next, have the student lie on a flat surface. While forcefully keeping the eye open, use clean cold water to gently rinse the eye. Irrigate the eye copiously for 20 minutes, everting the upper lid to flush the eye thoroughly. Next, discuss the situation with the student's parents after treating the student. Finally, arrange for transport to an emergency department where the student's eye can be further evaluated.

TEST-TAKING TIP: Visualize the steps prior to placing them in the correct order. The priority is to treat the student.

Content Area: Fundamentals; **Category of Health Alteration:** Safety, Disaster Preparedness, and Infection Control; **Integrated Processes:** Nursing Process Implementation; **Client Need:** Physiological Integrity/Physiological Adaptation/ Medical Emergencies; **Cognitive Level:** Application; **Reference:** Perry, S., Hockenberry, M., Lowdermilk, D., & Wilson, D. (2010), p. 1193.

81. ANSWER: 1, 3, 4, 5.
Closing the curtains provides for the client's privacy. Because the client is in a continuous seizure state, an oral airway is needed to ensure airway patency. However, it should be inserted when the client's jaw is relaxed to prevent injury. Clothing is loosened to prevent injury. Turning the client side-lying promotes the drainage of oral secretions, reducing the risk of aspiration. Restraining the client increases the risk for injury. Pillows and blankets help to avoid a traumatic injury.

TEST-TAKING TIP: Consider that status epilepticus is continuous seizures. Select options that include protecting the client's privacy, maintaining the client's airway, and protecting the client from injury.

Content Area: Fundamentals; **Category of Health Alteration:** Safety, Disaster Preparedness, and Infection Control; **Integrated Processes:** Nursing Process Implementation; **Client Need:** Safe and Effective Care Environment/Safety and Infection Control/Accident and Injury Prevention; **Cognitive Level:** Application; **Reference:** Potter, P., & Perry, A. (2009), p. 844.

82. A nurse is providing first aid to an unresponsive adult victim at the scene of an accident. Place the nurse's actions in numerical order (1–7).

_____ 1. Look, listen, and feel for breathing.

_____ 2. Cover the victim to prevent environmental exposure.

_____ 3. Open the victim's airway.

_____ 4. Palpate the carotid pulse and note whether it is present.

_____ 5. Ask others about the victim's allergies and medical history.

_____ 6. Complete a rapid baseline assessment of the victim's neurological status.

_____ 7. Check for other injuries.

83. A nurse is teaching a group of parents about the importance of encouraging their children to use bicycle helmets and about the legislation in some states requiring their use. Which findings, as a result of legislation, should the nurse note when teaching the parents? **Select all that apply.**

1. There has been a decrease in head injuries.
2. There has been a slight increase in helmet usage.
3. There has been no change in the use of helmets.
4. There has been no change in the safety of children.
5. Parental use of helmets has no impact on their children's use.

82. ANSWER: 4, 3, 1, 6, 7, 2, 5.
First palpate the carotid pulse and note whether it is present. If the pulse is present, then open the victim's airway and look, listen, and feel for breathing. Next complete a rapid baseline assessment of the client's neurological status and check for other injuries. Cover the victim to prevent environmental exposure. Finally, ask others about the victim's allergies and medical history, the last time of fluid or food ingestion, and events leading up to the injury.

TEST-TAKING TIP: Use the CABDEs (circulation, airway, breathing, disability, and exposure) of trauma assessment to prioritize actions.

Content Area: Fundamentals; **Category of Health Alteration:** Safety, Disaster Preparedness, and Infection Control; **Integrated Processes:** Nursing Process Implementation; **Client Need:** Physiological Integrity/Physiological Adaptation/ Medical Emergencies; **Cognitive Level:** Analysis; **Reference:** Field, J., Hazinski, M., Sayre, M., Chameides, L., Schexnayder, S., Hemphill, R., . . . Vander Howek, T. (2010) 2010 American Heart Association Guidelines for Cardiopulmonary Resuscitation and Emergency Cardiovascular Care Science. Part I: Executive Summary. Circulation, 122(18, Supp3), S640–S656, doi:10.1161CIRCULATION AHA.110.970889. Retrieved from http://circ.ahajournals.org/cgi/content/full/122/18_suppl_3/S640.

83. ANSWER: 1, 2.
There has been a decrease in head injuries and an increase in helmet usage. This is important for the safety of children as helmets protect the head from head injury. Usually, mandating a behavior will result in a better outcome of compliance and safety. Seeing a parent routinely wearing a helmet may well be a compelling reason for children to wear a helmet.

TEST-TAKING TIP: Note that options 3, 4, and 5 contain the words "no change" or "no impact."

Content Area: Fundamentals; **Category of Health Alteration:** Safety, Disaster Preparedness, and Infection Control; **Integrated Processes**: Teaching and Learning; **Client Need:** Safe and Effective Care Environment/Safety and Infection Control/ Accident and Injury Prevention; **Cognitive Level:** Analysis; **Reference:** Pillitteri, A. (2010), pp. 869–870. **EBP Reference:** Macpherson, A., & Spinks, A. (2007). Bicycle helmet legislation for the uptake of helmet use and prevention of head injuries. *Cochrane Database of Systematic Reviews, 2*, Art. No.: CD005401. DOI: 10.1002/ 14651858.CD005401.pub2. Retrieved from www.cochrane.org/reviews/en/ ab005401.html.

84. An experienced nurse observes a new nurse removing a gown and gloves after performing a wet-to-dry dressing change on a client who is in contact isolation. Based on the new nurse's action illustrated, which statement by the experienced nurse is correct?

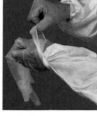

1. "Your gown should be removed before your contaminated gloves."
2. "You are using the correct procedure to remove your gloves and then your gown."
3. "During a wet-to-dry dressing change on a client in contact isolation, two pairs of gloves are always worn at the same time."
4. "Always discard the glove you removed first in the infectious waste before removing the other glove."

85. A nurse has been caring for a client in isolation with bacterial meningitis. The nurse is wearing personal protective equipment (PPE) that includes gown, gloves, and mask with eye shield. The nurse has completed the care and is leaving the client's room. In which sequence should the nurse remove the PPE? Place each step in the correct numerical order (1–4).

_____ 1. Untie the mask with eye shield, lowering the strings first. Remove mask avoiding touching the outside and discard. Repeat hand hygiene.

_____ 2. Untie the gown tied at the waist. Remove the first glove and hold it in the remaining gloved hand.

_____ 3. Perform hand hygiene. Grasp gown from inside at neck and pull gown down, roll up the soiled area to inside and discard.

_____ 4. Place fingers of ungloved hand inside cuff of second glove turning the glove inside out. Keep the first glove inside and then discard both gloves.

84. ANSWER: 2.

The new nurse is following the correct procedure in removing the contaminated gloves first because these would be more soiled than the gown. In order to remove the gown first, the new nurse would need to untie and grasp the gown with soiled gloves, risking skin exposure to contaminants on the gloves. It is unnecessary to wear two pairs of gloves at the same time. Two pairs of gloves should be used during a wet-to-dry procedure, one unsterile pair to remove the soiled dressing and a second sterile pair to cleanse, pack, and redress the wound. These, however, are not applied at the same time. To minimize exposure to contaminants and to use time efficiently, the first removed glove is held in the still-gloved hand and the second glove is slid over the first removed glove.

TEST-TAKING TIP: Select an option that both minimizes exposure to infectious waste and uses time efficiently.

Content Area: Fundamentals; **Category of Health Alteration:** Safety, Disaster Preparedness, and Infection Control; **Integrated Processes:** Nursing Process Evaluation; **Client Need:** Safe and Effective Care Environment/Safety and Infection Control/Standard Precautions/Transmission-Based Precautions/Surgical Asepsis; **Cognitive Level:** Analysis; **Reference:** Potter, P., & Perry, A. (2009), pp. 664–665.

85. ANSWER: 2, 4, 3, 1.

The nurse should untie the gown at the waist and proceed to remove the gloves. The nurse should then perform hand hygiene and proceed by removing the gown and then the mask. Hand hygiene should then be repeated.

TEST-TAKING TIP: Focus on the information in the question, visualize the process, and then proceed with listing the steps for removing PPE. Remember that the most contaminated item should be removed first.

Content Area: Fundamentals; **Category of Health Alteration:** Safety, Disaster Preparedness, and Infection Control; **Integrated Processes:** Nursing Process Implementation; **Client Need:** Safe and Effective Care Environment/Safety and Infection Control/Handling Hazardous and Infectious Materials; **Cognitive Level:** Application; **Reference:** Berman, A., Snyder, S., & McKinney, D. (2011), pp. 526–528.

Tab 3   Health Promotion and Maintenance | Childbearing Families

Test 8: Childbearing Families: Prenatal and Antepartal Management

86. A nurse performs Leopold's maneuver on a pregnant client who is 32 weeks gestation and determines that the fetus is left occiput anterior (LOA). When the nurse auscultates the fetal heart tones, at which location should the nurse expect the fetal heart tones to be the loudest? Place an X in the circled area where the fetal heart tones should be the loudest.

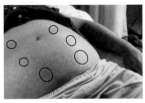

87. A nurse is planning care for a client during the first trimester of pregnancy. Which routine serology tests should the nurse plan to discuss with the client? **Select all that apply.**

1. Quadruple screen
2. Blood type and Rh status
3. Rapid plasma reagin (RPR)
4. Complete blood count (CBC)
5. Urinalysis

86. ANSWER:

When the fetus is left occiput-anterior, the fetal heart tones are best heard in the left lower quadrant.

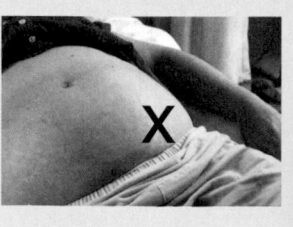

TEST-TAKING TIP: Read the question carefully. Note that the fetus is LOA. Eliminate all areas on the right side of the client's abdomen. Of the remaining options, think about the location of the fetal heart.

Content Area: Childbearing Families; **Category of Health Alteration:** Prenatal and Antepartal Management; **Integrated Processes:** Nursing Process Assessment; **Client Need:** Health Promotion and Maintenance/Ante/Intra/Postpartum and Newborn Care; **Cognitive Level:** Application; **Reference:** Ward, S., & Hisley, S. (2009), pp. 238–239.

87. ANSWER: 2, 3, 4.

Blood type and Rh status, RPR test for syphilis, and CBC are all standard screening tests that are routinely performed during the first trimester of pregnancy. The quadruple screen test is performed between 15 and 18 weeks in the second trimester. The quadruple screen test calculates the risk of a Down's syndrome, term pregnancy from maternal age, and the concentration of four markers in maternal blood (alpha-fetoprotein, unconjugated oestriol, human chorionic gonadotropin, and inhibin A) and is not a routine screening test. Although a urinalysis may be performed, it is not a serology test.

TEST-TAKING TIP: Eliminate the one test that is performed to calculate the risk of Down's syndrome. Then eliminate the test that is not a serology test.

Content Area: Childbearing Families; **Category of Health Alteration:** Prenatal and Antepartal Management; **Integrated Processes:** Nursing Process Planning; **Client Need:** Health Promotion and Maintenance/Health Screening; **Cognitive Level:** Application; **Reference:** Davidson, M., London, M., & Ladewig, P. (2008), pp. 547–548.

88. A nurse is caring for a woman who is being admitted for severe preeclampsia at 34 weeks gestation. The nurse is conducting the admission health history when the woman begins an eclamptic seizure. In which order should the nurse intervene when caring for this client? Place the nurse's actions in the correct numerical order (1–7).

_____ 1. Administer oxygen.

_____ 2. Suction oral secretions as needed.

_____ 3. Position the client in the left lateral position.

_____ 4. Clear the client's airway.

_____ 5. Obtain intravenous access by inserting a 16- or 18-gauge catheter.

_____ 6. Administer magnesium sulfate per protocol.

_____ 7. Call for immediate assistance.

89. A nurse is counseling a pregnant woman diagnosed with gestational diabetes (GDM) at 28.5 weeks. Which information should the nurse discuss with the client? **Select all that apply.**

1. Weekly nonstress test beginning at 32–34 weeks
2. Amniocentesis at this time
3. Induction at 36 weeks gestation
4. Nutritional counseling with a dietician
5. Delivery before expected date of conception (EDC)

88. ANSWER: 7, 4, 1, 2, 3, 5, 6.

Because this is an emergency situation, the nurse should first call for help. The airway should be cleared and oxygen should be administered. The nurse should provide oral suctioning as needed to maintain the airway. The woman should be placed in a left lateral position to facilitate blood flow to the uterus and the fetus. Once the airway is stabilized, an intravenous line should be started, and magnesium sulfate should be administered.

TEST-TAKING TIP: Use the ABCs to determine the proper sequencing of the nurse's actions in this emergency situation. Calling for help should be the first step in any emergency situation.

Content Area: Childbearing Families; **Category of Health Alteration:** Prenatal and Antepartal Management; **Integrated Processes:** Nursing Process Implementation; **Client Need:** Physiological Integrity/Physiological Adaptation/Alterations in Body Systems; **Cognitive Level:** Application; **Reference:** Pillitteri, A. (2010), pp. 578–579.

89. ANSWER: 1, 4, 5.

Because gestational diabetes can result in delayed lung maturity and complications, the nurse should discuss nonstress testing, nutritional counseling with a dietician, and delivery before her due date. There is no indication for amniocentesis. Induction is not indicated until at least 38 weeks.

TEST-TAKING TIP: Recall that the normal gestation period is between 38 and 42 weeks. Eliminate options that would prevent further lung maturity.

Content Area: Childbearing Families; **Category of Health Alteration:** Prenatal and Antepartal Management; **Integrated Processes:** Teaching and Learning; **Client Need:** Health Promotion and Maintenance/Ante/Intra/Postpartum and Newborn Care; **Cognitive Level:** Analysis; **Reference:** Pillitteri, A. (2010), pp. 536–538; **EBP Reference:** American Dietetic Association (ADA). (2008). Gestational diabetes mellitus (GDM). Evidence based nutrition practice guideline. Chicago (IL): American Dietetic Association (ADA). Retrieved from www.guideline .gov/content.aspx?id=14888&search=maternal+nutrition.

90. A client who is 39 weeks pregnant presents for her routine prenatal appointment. Which signs should suggest to the nurse that the client is experiencing preeclampsia? **Select all that apply.**

1. Blood pressure (BP) 144/94 mm Hg
2. Proteinuria 3.8 grams in a 24-hour urine
3. 330 mL of urine in 24 hours
4. Platelet count 152,000/mm³
5. Chronic heartburn

91. A nurse is teaching a woman diagnosed with placenta previa at 35 weeks gestation. The nurse uses a diagram to teach the client. At which location should the nurse show the woman that the placenta previa is occurring? Place an X at the appropriate location on the illustration.

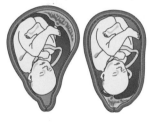

90. ANSWER: 1, 2, 3.

The normal BP should be less than 140/90 mm Hg during pregnancy. There should be less than 3 grams of protein in a 24-hour urine, and the volume should be greater than 500 mL in a 24-hour period. A platelet count between 150,000 and 450,000/mm^3 is within the normal range. Heartburn is common in the third trimester and is not a definitive sign of preeclampsia, but should be evaluated to rule out epigastric pain.

TEST-TAKING TIP: Review normal values and select the values that are abnormal. Remember chronic heartburn can occur with many disorders and should be eliminated.

Content Area: Childbearing Families; **Category of Health Alteration:** Prenatal and Antepartal Management; **Integrated Processes:** Nursing Process Assessment; **Client Need:** Physiological Integrity/Reduction of Risk Potential/Potential for Complications from Surgical Procedures and Health Alterations; **Cognitive Level:** Analysis; **Reference:** Pillitteri, A. (2010), pp. 575–577.

91. ANSWER:

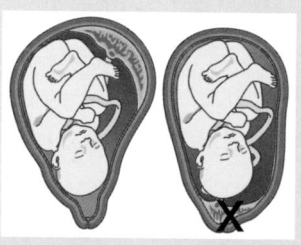

Placenta previa is present where the placenta is covering the cervical os.

TEST-TAKING TIP: Focus on the illustration and the location of the placenta.

Content Area: Childbearing Families; **Category of Health Alteration:** Prenatal and Antepartal Management; **Integrated Processes:** Teaching and Learning; **Client Need:** Physiological Integrity/Physiological Adaptation/Alterations in Body Systems; **Cognitive Level:** Application; **Reference:** Chapman, L., & Durham, R. F. (2010), pp. 117–118.

92. A client who is 32 weeks pregnant is prescribed a daily iron supplement to treat iron deficiency anemia. A nurse is teaching the client about foods and fluids that enhance the absorption of the iron supplement. Which foods and fluids identified by the client as enhancing the absorption of the iron supplement suggests to the nurse that the teaching has been effective? **Select all that apply.**

1. Pineapple juice
2. Liver
3. Oranges
4. Spinach
5. Legumes

93. An experienced nurse is teaching a new nurse how to perform fetal movement counts. Which statements about fetal movement assessment should be included in the instructions to the new nurse? **Select all that apply.**

1. Fetal movement counts should be initiated once the woman perceives fetal movement.
2. Glucose consumption is not associated with fetal movement.
3. A reduction of fetal activity is commonly associated with chronic conditions and not nonreassuring fetal status.
4. A decrease in fetal movement can occur as a result of fetal sleep patterns.
5. Teach the pregnant client to notify the health care provider (HCP) if there are fewer than 10 movements in 3 hours.

92. ANSWER: 1, 3.

Because iron is best absorbed from an acid medium, pineapple juice or oranges will enhance its absorption. Liver, spinach, and legumes are iron-rich foods. These will not enhance the absorption of the iron supplement.

TEST-TAKING TIP: The focus of the question is on enhancing the absorption of the iron supplement. Read the question carefully and eliminate the foods that are high in iron.

Content Area: Childbearing Families; **Category of Health Alteration:** Prenatal and Antepartal Management; **Integrated Processes:** Nursing Process Evaluation; **Client Need:** Health Promotion and Maintenance/Ante/Intra/Postpartum and Newborn Care; **Cognitive Level:** Application; **Reference:** Pillitteri, A. (2010), pp. 521–523; **EBP Reference:** U.S. Preventive Services Task Force (USPSTF). (2006). Screening for iron deficiency anemia—including iron supplementation for children and pregnant women. Rockville (MD): Agency for Healthcare Research and Quality (AHRQ). Retrieved from www.guideline.gov/content.aspx?id=9274.

93. ANSWER: 2, 3, 4, 5.

Glucose intake does not affect fetal movement patterns. A reduction in fetal activity is typically associated with chronic conditions, such as placental insufficiency, rather than an acute, nonreassuring fetal status heart rate pattern. Fetal activity can be affected by the sleep cycles of the fetus. Most women feel fetal movement at least 10 times in 3 hours; fewer than that may indicate fetal distress. Fetal movement counts should be initiated at 28 weeks gestation.

TEST-TAKING TIP: Eliminate any incorrect options. Review the pathophysiology of fetal movement to determine the best possible option.

Content Area: Childbearing Families; **Category of Health Alteration:** Prenatal and Antepartal Management; **Integrated Processes:** Teaching and Learning; **Client Need:** Health Promotion and Maintenance/Ante/Intra/Postpartum and Newborn Care **Cognitive level:** Application; **Reference:** Davidson, M., London, M., & Ladewig, P. (2008), pp. 385, 551; **EBP Reference:** Antenatal fetal surveillance. (2007). In: Fetal health surveillance: antepartum and intrapartum consensus guideline. *Journal of Obstetrics and Gynaecology Canada 2007, 29*(9 Suppl 4), S9–23.

94. A client who is pregnant is experiencing frequent backaches. Which position should a nurse recommend to help the client relieve her backache?

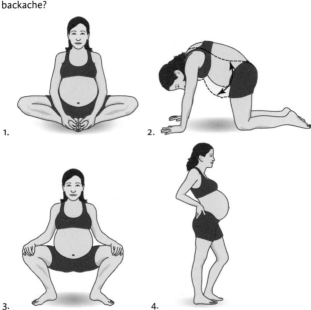

1.

2.

3.

4.

94. ANSWER: 2.
Pelvic rocking helps relieve backache during pregnancy. In pelvic rocking, the woman hollows her back and then arches it. Illustration 1 is tailor sitting and is used to strengthen the thighs and stretch the perineal muscles to make them supple. Illustration 3 is squatting and is used to stretch the muscles of the pelvic floor. Illustration 4 is hyperextension of the lower back and should be avoided to prevent muscle strain.

TEST-TAKING TIP: First, eliminate the one illustration that would increase muscle strain. Then, focus on eliminating the illustrations that would enhance strengthening the thighs, stretching the perineal muscles, and pelvic stretching.

Content Area: Childbearing Families; **Category of Health Alteration:** Prenatal and Antepartal Management; **Integrated Processes:** Caring; Nursing Process Implementation; **Client Need:** Health Promotion and Maintenance/Ante/Intra/Postpartum and Newborn Care; **Cognitive Level:** Application; **Reference:** Pillitteri, A. (2010), pp. 328–329.

Test 9: Childbearing Families: Intrapartal Management

95. A nurse observes the fetal heart rate (FHR) pattern illustrated. Which documentation by the nurse is correct?

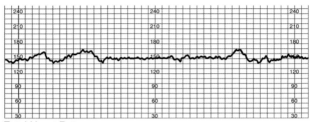

Fetal Heart Rate

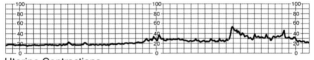

Uterine Contractions

1. Electronic fetal monitoring shows fetal heart rate (FHR) accelerations with uterine contractions.
2. Electronic fetal monitoring shows a normal FHR baseline with no change in response to contractions.
3. Electronic fetal monitoring shows FHR early decelerations in response to uterine contractions.
4. Electronic fetal monitoring shows FHR late decelerations in response to uterine contractions.

95. ANSWER: 1.
The illustration shows fetal heart rate accelerations in the top graph and uterine contractions in the bottom graph. Acceleration is an increase in the FHR of 15 bpm above the FHR baseline that lasts for at least 15 to 30 seconds. Option 2 is incorrect because the FHR increases in response to uterine contractions. With FHR decelerations, options 3 and 4, there would be a decrease in FHR below the baseline FHR in response to uterine contractions.

TEST-TAKING TIP: The term "acceleration" refers to an increase in FHR and "deceleration" refers to a decrease in FHR. Use this information to eliminate options.

Content Area: Childbearing Families; **Category of Health Alteration:** Intrapartal Management; **Integrated Processes:** Communication and Documentation; **Client Need:** Health Promotion and Maintenance/Ante/Intra/Postpartum and Newborn Care; **Cognitive Level:** Application; **Reference:** Ward, S., & Hisley, S. (2009), pp. 382–383.

96. A client is to have a repeat cesarean birth in the operating room. Which actions should the nurse include when planning care for this client? **Select all that apply.**

1. Position the woman in a supine position.
2. Provide oxygen via nasal cannula.
3. Initiate intravenous access.
4. Monitor maternal vital signs.
5. Assess the fetal heart rate for the final time before entering the operative suite.
6. Administer intravenous anesthesia as needed.

97. An experienced nurse determines that a new nurse intervenes appropriately in various intrapartal situations by placing a fetal scalp electrode for electronic fetal monitoring. Which situations prompted the experienced nurse's conclusion? **Select all that apply.**

1. A client with cervical dilation to 2 centimeters
2. A client with effacement to 50%
3. A client with ruptured membranes
4. The ability to reach the presenting part
5. A client with multiple gestation

96. ANSWER: 2, 3, 4.
The role of the nurse includes providing oxygen via nasal cannula, initiating intravenous access, and monitoring maternal vital signs. The client should be placed in a left lateral tilt position so that fetal oxygenation is maximized, and the fetal heart rate should be monitored every 5 minutes until the time the sterile abdominal preparation is completed. An anesthesiologist or nurse anesthetist administers anesthesia. This is not a nursing responsibility.

TEST-TAKING TIP: Apply knowledge of spinal anesthesia and the major responsibilities that the nurse performs in preparation for its administration.

Content Area: Childbearing Families; **Category of Health Alteration:** Intrapartal Management; **Integrated Processes:** Nursing Process Planning; **Client Need:** Physiological Integrity/Reduction of Risk Potential/Potential for Complications from Surgical Procedures and Health Alterations; **Cognitive Level:** Application; **Reference:** Davidson, M., London, M., & Ladewig, P. (2008), pp. 707–708.

97. ANSWER: 1, 3, 4, 5.
Cervical dilation to 2 centimeters, ruptured membranes, ability to reach the presenting part, and multiple gestation are indications for placement of a fetal scalp electrode for internal monitoring of the fetus. Cervical effacement is not a crucial factor in placement of an internal monitor.

TEST-TAKING TIP: Identify the proper situations for placing internal monitors. Select options that include fetal factors, maternal factors, uterine factors, and complications of pregnancy.

Content Area: Childbearing Families; **Category of Health Alteration:** Intrapartal Management; **Integrated Processes:** Nursing Process Evaluation; **Client Need:** Physiological Integrity/Reduction of Risk Potential/Potential for Complications from Surgical Procedures and Health Alterations; **Cognitive level:** Application; **Reference:** Davidson, M., London, M., & Ladewig, P. (2008), p. 626.

98. A nurse is assisting with the administration of a continuous lumbar epidural block for pain control for a laboring client. After explaining the procedure to the client, what is the correct sequence for the nurse's actions? Place each action in the correct numerical order (1–6).

_____ 1. Position the client in a semireclining position with a left lateral tilt for 10 minutes.

_____ 2. Monitor the blood pressure every 2 minutes for 10 minutes.

_____ 3. Position the client on her side with her knees slightly flexed and remain beside her.

_____ 4. Assist the client to turn from side to side every hour.

_____ 5. Ask the client to void.

_____ 6. Administer 1,000 mL of intravenous (IV) Ringer's lactate solution over 30 minutes as ordered.

99. A nurse's laboring client states that she feels intense pressure and cannot stop pushing with the contractions despite the fact that she is only 8 centimeters dilated. Which parameters should the nurse monitor when caring for this client? **Select all that apply.**

1. Cervical edema
2. Hypercontractility of the uterus
3. Bruising of the cervix
4. Retardation of dilation
5. Slowing of labor progression

98. ANSWER: 5, 6, 3, 1, 2, 4.
First ask the client to void before the procedure begins because urinary retention is a side effect of epidural analgesia. The most common complication of an epidural block is maternal hypotension. This can be prevented by preloading with a rapid infusion of IV fluids. For insertion of the epidural catheter the client should be positioned on her side with knees slightly flexed. This position allows access to the epidural space. The nurse should stand beside the client to assist her to maintain the correct position. After the medication has been injected, the client should be positioned in a semireclining position with a lateral tilt to allow for distribution of the block. Tilting the client to the side will eliminate the risk of developing supine hypotensive syndrome. Because of the risk of hypotension the client's blood pressure should be monitored frequently (per agency policy). Turning the client from side to side once the block has been established will prevent a one-sided block.

TEST-TAKING TIP: Think through the logical progression of the steps that would be necessary when assisting with epidural analgesia administration.

Content Area: Childbearing Families; **Category of Health Alteration:** Intrapartal Management; **Integrated Processes:** Nursing Process Implementation; **Client Need:** Physiological Integrity/Pharmacological and Parenteral Therapies/Pharmacological Pain Management; **Cognitive Level:** Analysis; **References:** Davidson, M., London, M., & Ladewig, P. (2008), pp. 317, 694, 697–698, 701; Potter, P., & Perry, A. (2009), p. 354.

99. ANSWER: 1, 3, 4, 5.
Early bearing down during the first stage, before the cervix has fully dilated, can cause cervical edema, bruising of the cervix, retardation of dilation, and a slowing of labor progression. Bearing down has implications for the cervix but does not affect uterine contractility because contractions are involuntary.

TEST-TAKING TIP: Consider the etiology of early bearing down and how such bearing down could affect the cervix. Eliminate an option that affects the uterus since contractions are involuntary.

Content Area: Childbearing Families; **Category of Health Alteration:** Intrapartal Management; **Integrated Processes:** Nursing Process Analysis; **Client Need:** Physiological Integrity/Reduction of Risk Potential/Potential for Complications from Surgical Procedures and Health Alterations; **Cognitive level:** Application; **Reference:** Ward, S., & Hisley, S. (2009), p. 359.

100. A nurse is caring for a client who just received an epidural anesthetic in preparation for a cesarean birth. The client's blood pressure prior to the epidural anesthetic was 112/72 mm Hg and is now 78/42 mm Hg. Which measures should the nurse implement? **Select all that apply.**

1. Administer intravenous fluids.
2. Encourage oral fluids.
3. Initiate leg compressions.
4. Administer epinephrine.
5. Assist the client to a sitting position.

101. A nurse is caring for a laboring client who is now 5 centimeters dilated and is requesting an epidural for pain relief. Upon the nurse's review of the client's laboratory report, which finding should be considered as a contraindication for the regional anesthesia?

Serum Laboratory Test	Client's Value
RBC	4.1 cells/mcL
WBC	10,420 cells/mcL
MCH	25 pg/cell
MCHC	28.2 gm/dL
MCV	78 fetoliter
Hgb	11.1 g/dL
Hct	33.4%
PLT	48,000/mm^3

1. White blood cells (WBC)
2. Red blood cells (RBC)
3. Hematocrit (HCT)
4. Platelets (PLT)

100. ANSWER: 1, 3, 4.
The client is experiencing hypotension from the use of spinal anesthesia. Intravenous fluids, leg compression, and administration of epinephrine are all associated with successful management of hypotension. Oral hydration is contraindicated for a woman undergoing a cesarean birth because it can increase the risk of aspiration during surgery. Placing the client in a sitting position with the intent of preventing upward spread of the hyperbaric solution is dangerous because it will cause venous pooling in the lower extremities, further decreasing the maternal blood pressure.

TEST-TAKING TIP: Consider that the client is to undergo a surgical procedure, thus eliminate option 2. Consider the effects of blood pooling when a hypotensive client is positioned in a sitting position and eliminate option 5.

Content Area: Childbearing Families; **Category of Health Alteration:** Intrapartal Management; **Integrated Processes:** Nursing Process Implementation; **Client Need:** Physiological Integrity/Reduction of Risk Potential/Potential for Complications from Surgical Procedures and Health Alterations; **Cognitive level:** Analysis; **Reference:** Davidson, M., London, M., & Ladewig, P. (2008), p. 707; **EBP Reference:** Cyna, A., Andrew, M., Emmett, R., Middleton, P., Simmons, S. (2006). Techniques for preventing hypotension during spinal anesthesia for cesarean section. *Cochrane Database of Systematic Reviews 2001, 3.* Art. No.: CD002251. DOI: 10.1002/14651858.CD002251. pub2. Retrieved from www.cochrane.org/reviews/en/ab002251.html.

101. ANSWER: 4.
Platelets less than 100,000/mm³ are considered abnormal. Platelet counts below 50,000/mm³ are a contraindication for regional anesthesia because it increases the client's risk for bleeding. The WBC, RBC, and HCT levels can be slightly abnormal in labor and pregnancy; however, these levels would not be a contraindication for regional anesthesia.

TEST-TAKING TIP: Select the abnormal laboratory value that would increase the client's risk for bleeding.

Content Area: Childbearing Families; **Category of Health Alteration:** Intrapartal Management; **Integrated Processes:** Nursing Process Assessment; **Client Need:** Physiological Integrity/Physiological Adaptation/Alterations in Body Systems; **Cognitive Level:** Analysis; **Reference:** Chapman, L., & Durham, R. F. (2010), p. 225.

Test 10: Childbearing Families: Postpartal Management

102. A nurse is assessing the condition of a client's midline episiotomy. Place an X at the location on the illustration where the nurse should assess the midline episiotomy.

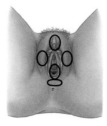

103. A nurse assesses a postpartal client who is 18 hours post-vaginal delivery and gathers the following information: *Blood pressure (BP), 110/60 mm Hg; pulse, 65 beats per minute; respirations, 20 breaths per minute; temperature, 102.2°F (39°C); cramping pain rated 4 out of 10 on a 0 to 10 pain scale; foul-smelling lochia and chills.* Based on this information, in which order should the nurse complete the following actions? Place each action in the correct numerical order (1–5).

_____ 1. Assist with ambulation to promote uterine drainage.
_____ 2. Encourage the client to increase her fluid intake.
_____ 3. Notify the health care provider (HCP).
_____ 4. Administer the prescribed ibuprofen (Motrin) 600 mg oral.
_____ 5. Document administering the medication and the physical findings.

102. ANSWER:
The lowest circled area should have been selected. A midline episiotomy is performed along the median raphe of the perineum. It extends down from the vaginal orifice to the fiber of the rectal sphincter.

TEST-TAKING TIP: Use the term "midline" to assist in determining the location on the perineum.

Content Area: Childbearing Families; **Category of Health Alteration:** Postpartal Management; **Integrated Processes:** Nursing Process Assessment; **Client Need:** Health Promotion and Maintenance/Techniques of Physical Assessment; **Cognitive Level:** Application; **Reference:** Davidson, M., London, M., & Ladewig, P. (2008), p. 775.

103. ANSWER: 3, 4, 5, 2, 1.
First the nurse should notify the HCP. The symptoms suggest that the client has endometritis. Laboratory tests and antibiotics are likely to be prescribed. Next administer ibuprofen. Because of its anti-inflammatory effect, many HCPs order a nonsteroidal anti-inflammatory medication (NSAID) to serve as an antipyretic and analgesic. The medication should be documented after administration. If the nurse has not already documented the physical findings, this should be completed while the nurse is using the chart. Next, the nurse should encourage the client to increase her fluid intake to maintain hydration because an elevated temperature increases fluid loss. Although ambulation will promote uterine drainage, rest should be encouraged initially. Only after the temperature is reduced, pain is controlled, and antibiotics are initiated, would the client be ready to ambulate.

TEST-TAKING TIP: Consider that the client may be experiencing endometritis. Use Maslow's Hierarchy of Needs theory to place items in the correct sequence.

Content Area: Childbearing Families; **Category of Health Alteration:** Postpartal Management; **Integrated Processes:** Nursing Process Implementation; **Client Need:** Physiological Integrity/Physiological Adaptation/Alterations in Body Systems; **Cognitive Level:** Analysis; **Reference:** Whitehead, D., Weiss, S., & Tappen, R. (2010), pp. 520–521.

104. A postpartal client who has chosen to bottle feed her infant has developed painful breast engorgement. Which actions should a nurse plan to recommend for this client? **Select all that apply.**

1. Apply ice to her painful breasts.
2. Express the milk from her breasts every 2 hours.
3. Take ibuprofen (Motrin) for pain control.
4. Wear a sports bra continuously until the pain is gone.
5. Shower and allow the warm water to run on her sore breasts.

105. A nurse is assessing the location of the fundus of a client who is 8 days postpartum. Place an X on the abdomen where the nurse should expect to locate the client's fundus.

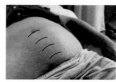

104. ANSWER: 1, 3, 4.
Ice reduces milk production and decreases breast heaviness. Anti-inflammatory drugs have been shown to significantly improve discomfort associated with engorgement. Wearing a supportive bra mechanically suppresses lactation. Any type of breast stimulation will increase milk production. Clients should be advised to let shower water flow over their backs and avoid direct stimulation of the breasts to decrease engorgement.

TEST-TAKING TIP: Eliminate options that will increase engorgement or breast milk production and not relieve pain.

Content Area: Childbearing Families; **Category of Health Alteration:** Postpartal Management; **Integrated Processes:** Caring; Teaching and Learning; **Client Need:** Health Promotion and Maintenance/Ante/Intra/Postpartum and Newborn Care; **Cognitive Level:** Application; **References:** Davidson, M., London, M., & Ladewig, P. (2008), pp. 1081–1082; Perry, S., Hockenberry, M., Lowdermilk, D., & Wilson, D. (2010), pp. 694–697.

105. ANSWER:
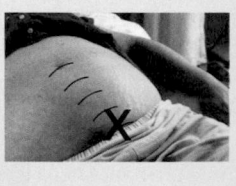
Within an hour after birth the uterus is at the level of the umbilicus and then descends at a rate of about 1 cm/day (one fingerbreadth). About the 8th day the uterus is just below the symphysis pubis. After 10 days, the uterus has fully descended into the pelvis and is no longer palpable.

TEST-TAKING TIP: The usual rate of descent is 1 cm/day, and the space between each line in the illustration is approximately 2 fingerbreadths (2 cm). Use this information to select the correct option.

Content Area: Childbearing Families; **Category of Health Alteration:** Postpartal Management; **Integrated Processes:** Nursing Process Assessment; **Client Need:** Health Promotion and Maintenance/Ante/Intra/Postpartum and Newborn Care; **Cognitive Level:** Application; **Reference:** Ward, S., & Hisley, S. (2009), pp. 475–476.

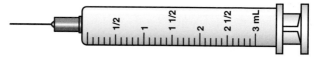

106. Which interventions should a nurse plan to enhance comfort and promote healing of a client's episiotomy? **Select all that apply.**

1. Look for discoloration of the client's perineum.
2. Ask about the client's need to defecate.
3. Prepare a tub filled with 4–6 inches of warm water and assist the client with a sitz bath.
4. Teach the client to apply a few drops of tea tree oil from a prefilled applicator to the wound.
5. Inform the client that the episiotomy sutures are absorbable and will not need to be removed.
6. Apply heat to the client's abdomen.

107. A nurse is preparing to administer methylergonovine (Methergine) 200 mcg IV to prevent postpartum hemorrhage caused by a client's uterine atony. The medication is supplied in a 1-mL ampule with 0.2 mg/mL. Place an X on the syringe to indicate the correct amount of medication that the nurse should prepare for administration.

106. ANSWER: 3, 4.
Sitz baths are used to relieve pain, itching, or muscle spasms. Tea tree oil has anti-inflammatory properties and is believed to be beneficial in facilitating healing of the episiotomy site. Looking for perineal discoloration or asking about the need to defecate are assessments for perineal hematoma and not interventions. Teaching that the sutures are absorbable, while important, does not enhance comfort and promote healing. Heat should not be applied to the abdomen because of the potential for uterine relaxation and bleeding.

TEST-TAKING TIP: Carefully read the question and eliminate options that are assessments and not interventions. Of the interventions, eliminate any that will not promote comfort and healing.

Content Area: Childbearing Families; **Category of Health Alteration:** Postpartal Management; **Integrated Processes:** Nursing Process Planning; **Client Need:** Health Promotion and Maintenance/Ante/Intra/Postpartum and Newborn Care; **Cognitive Level:** Analysis; **Reference:** Ward, S., & Hisley, S. (2009), pp. 478–479.

107. ANSWER:

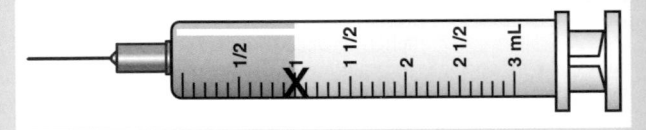

First, convert mcg to mg: 1,000 mcg: 1 mg :: 200 mcg : *X* mg

1,000 *X* = 200   *X* = 0.2 mg

Then, determine the amount to withdraw: 0.2 mg = 1 mL.

TEST-TAKING TIP: Convert microgram to milligram (1,000 mcg = 1 mg)

Content Area: Childbearing Families; **Category of Health Alteration:** Postpartal Management; **Integrated Processes:** Nursing Process Implementation; **Client Need:** Physiological Integrity/Pharmacological and Parenteral Therapies/Dosage Calculation; **Cognitive Level:** Application; **References:** Deglin, J., Vallerand, A., & Sanoski, C. (2011), p. 842; Pickar, G., & Abernethy, A. (2008), p. 46; Ward, S., & Hisley, S. (2009), p. 478.

108. A nurse is conversing with a client who delivered vaginally 48 hours previously. Which statements indicate that the client needs education on sexual activity following childbirth? **Select all that apply.**

1. "If my spouse and I have sexual intercourse in about 2 weeks, the risk for infection is minimal."
2. "I told my husband that the male on top position may be more comfortable for me during sexual intercourse."
3. "Because of the hormonal changes, my husband and I can expect that our sexual experience and my orgasm will be more intense than before the pregnancy."
4. "My husband and I should delay having intercourse until my vaginal discharge has stopped."
5. "Due to hormonal changes, I may need vaginal lubrication for comfort prior to intercourse."
6. "We plan to use contraceptives because I was told in the education classes that I could get pregnant even though I just had a baby."

109. A nurse is weighing the perineal pads for a client who has had increased vaginal bleeding despite uterine massage to prevent bleeding. The client has six saturated pads in the past 1 hour, each weighing 90 grams after subtracting the dry weight of the pads. How many milliliters (mL) of blood did the client lose in the last hour?

_____mL (Record your answer as a whole number.)

108. ANSWER: 2, 3.

To avoid discomfort, a position in which the female has control of the depth of penile penetration, such as side-lying or female on top, is recommended for the initial sexual experiences. Due to hormonal alterations the sexual experience and the orgasm may be less intense (not more intense) than before the pregnancy. The risk of infection is minimal by 2 weeks postpartum; however, the presence of lochia discharge indicates that healing is not yet complete. Therefore, the client should delay first intercourse until the vaginal discharge has stopped. Vaginal dryness may be present in the postpartal period because of low estrogen levels. The woman may need external lubrication until estrogen levels have returned to prepregnancy levels. According to research, postpartum education about contraception use led to more contraception use and fewer unplanned pregnancies.

TEST-TAKING TIP: The key phrase is "needs education." Select options that are incorrect statements.

Content Area: Childbearing Families; **Category of Health Alteration:** Postpartal Management; **Integrated Processes:** Nursing Process Evaluation; **Client Need:** Health Promotion and Maintenance/Ante/Intra/Postpartum and Newborn Care; **Cognitive Level:** Application; **Reference:** Pillitteri, A. (2010), pp. 441–442, 437–438; **EBP Reference:** Lopez L. M., Hiller, J. E., & Grimes, D. A. (2010). Education for contraceptive use by women after childbirth. *Cochrane Database of Systematic Reviews* 2010, 1, Art. No.: CD001863. DOI: 10.1002/14651858.CD001863.pub2. Retrieved from www.cochrane.org/reviews/en/ab001863.html.

109. ANSWER: 540

Six pads × 90 grams = 540 grams. One gram of weight is equal to one milliliter of blood.

TEST-TAKING TIP: Use the conversion: 1 mL = 1 gram.

Content Area: Childbearing Families; **Category of Health Alteration:** Postpartal Management; **Integrated Processes:** Nursing Process Analysis; **Client Need:** Physiological Integrity/Physiological Adaptation/Medical Emergencies; **Cognitive Level:** Application; **Reference:** Davidson, M., London, M., & Ladewig, P. (2008), p. 1164; **EBP Reference:** Hofmeyr, G., Abdel-Aleem, H., & Abdel-Aleem, M. (2008). Uterine massage for preventing postpartum haemorrhage. *Cochrane Database of Systematic Reviews* 2008, 3, Art. No.: CD006431. DOI: 10.1002/14651858. CD006431.pub2. Retrieved from www.cochrane.org/reviews/en/ab006431.html

Test 11: Childbearing Families: Neonatal and High Risk Neonatal Management

110. A nurse is performing an initial newborn assessment. Following the assessment, which findings should prompt the nurse to inform the health care provider (HCP)? **Select all that apply.**

1. Cleft lip
2. Positive Babinski reflex
3. Strabismus
4. Heart rate 94
5. Respiration 26

111. A nurse is preparing to collect blood from a neonate for newborn screening tests. Which location should the nurse use to obtain the blood sample?

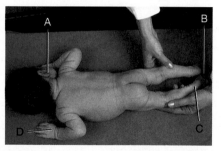

1. Location A
2. Location B
3. Location C
4. Location D

110. ANSWER: 1, 4, 5.
The HCP should be informed about abnormal findings. A facial anomaly of the lip or pallet or a heart rate less than 100 with respirations of 26 are abnormal findings. Newborn screening for cystic fibrosis should be considered. Assessing a positive Babinski and strabismus are considered normal newborn assessment findings.

TEST-TAKING TIP: Consider that the normal respiratory rate of a term neonate is 30–60 breaths per minute and the heart rate 120–160 beats per minute when selecting the correct options.

Content Area: Childbearing Families; **Category of Health Alteration:** Neonatal and High Risk Neonatal Management; **Integrated Processes:** Nursing Process Assessment; **Client Need:** Health Promotion and Maintenance/Ante/Intra/Postpartum and Newborn Care; **Cognitive Level:** Analysis; **Reference:** Kyle, T. (2008), p. 533; **EBP Reference:** Southern, K., Mérelle, M., Dankert-Roelse, J., & Nagelkerke A. (2009). Newborn screening for cystic fibrosis. *Cochrane Database of Systematic Reviews*, Issue 1, Art. No.: CD001402. DOI: 10.1002/14651858.CD001402. pub2. Retrieved from www.cochrane.org/reviews/en/ab001402.html.

111. ANSWER: 3.
The heel is used for performing a heelstick to obtain blood for screening tests. The area is easily accessible, and circulation to the peripheral area can be enhanced by warming the foot with a warm, moist washcloth. There is less blood flow to the ear lobes and big toe of a neonate and they are not the areas of choice. It is unnecessary to obtain blood from the hand veins.

TEST-TAKING TIP: Think about the area that has the largest exposure area for performing the needle-stick.

Content Area: Childbearing Families; **Category of Health Alteration:** Neonatal and High Risk Neonatal Management; **Integrated Processes:** Nursing Process Implementation; **Client Need:** Health Promotion and Maintenance/Ante/Intra/Postpartum and Newborn Care; **Cognitive Level:** Application; **Reference:** Chapman, L., & Durham, R. F. (2010), p. 305.

112. A nurse is planning care for a male newborn infant who has increased serum bilirubin levels and is receiving phototherapy. Which interventions should the nurse include in the plan of care? **Select all that apply.**

1. Cover the infant's eyes with eye patches while under phototherapy lights.
2. Reposition the infant every 2 hours.
3. Dress the infant in a diaper and T-shirt at all times.
4. Keep the infant under the light during feedings.
5. Increase the infant's fluid intake by 25%.
6. Weigh the infant daily.

113. A nurse evaluates that the urine output is normal during an 8-hour shift for a pre-term infant weighing 4 pounds. The infant had four diapers that weighed 10 grams, 8 grams, 11 grams, and 9 grams after the dry weight of the diaper was subtracted. How many milliliters (mL) should the nurse have calculated for the total amount of urine the newborn voided during the 8-hour shift?

_____ mL (Record your answer as a whole number.)

112. ANSWER: 1, 2, 5, 6.
Covering the infant's eyes during phototherapy protects the retina from damage due to high-intensity light. Repositioning the infant every 2 hours provides equal exposure of all skin areas and prevents pressure areas. Providing extra fluid replaces fluid lost due to watery stools, a common side effect of phototherapy. Daily weights help monitor intake and output. Weighing the infant daily also monitors for dehydration, which may occur as a result of loose stools and increased insensible water loss. Weighing the infant daily also monitors for possible fluid overload from intravenous fluids. The infant should have minimal coverage (diaper area only) to provide maximal skin exposure to phototherapy. To provide visual and tactile stimulation and to promote parent-infant attachment, the infant should be removed from the phototherapy and the eye shield removed during feedings.

TEST-TAKING TIP: Consider that phototherapy changes bilirubin in peripheral circulation so it can easily be eliminated from the body. Therefore as much of the skin surface as possible must be exposed to the treatment. Thus, eliminate option 3.

Content Area: Childbearing Families; **Category of Health Alteration:** Neonatal and High-Risk Neonatal Management; **Integrated Processes:** Nursing Process Planning; **Client Need:** Physiological Integrity/Reduction of Risk Potential/Therapeutic Procedures; **Cognitive Level:** Application; **Reference:** Davidson, M., London, M., & Ladewig, P. (2008), pp. 1014–1016.

113. ANSWER: 38
Add the weight of the diapers (10 + 8 + 11 + 9 = 38). Use the equivalent, 1 g = 1 mL. A preterm infant weighing 4 pounds (1.8 kg) should have an output of 1 to 3 mL/kg per hour or 14.4 to 43.2 mL per 8 hours.

TEST-TAKING TIP: Use the equivalent 1 g dry weight = 1 mL to calculate the correct amount.

Content Area: Childbearing Families; **Category of Health Alteration:** Neonatal and High Risk Neonatal Management; **Integrated Processes:** Nursing Process Evaluation; **Client Need:** Physiological Integrity/Basic Care and Comfort/Elimination; **Cognitive Level:** Application; **References:** Davidson, M., London, M., & Ladewig, P. (2008), p. 955; Ward, S., Ward. S., & Hisley, S. (2009), p. 631.

114. A nurse is documenting after suctioning an infant's nasal passages. In which order should the nurse document the statements? Place the statements in the correct numerical order (1–6).

_____ 1. Both nares suctioned with bulb syringe.

_____ 2. Small amount of clear thick mucus draining from both nares.

_____ 3. Suctioning produced small amount of clear thick mucus.

_____ 4. Procedure tolerated and respirations returned to normal rate.

_____ 5. Respirations 62 per minute, breathing without difficulty, and no retractions noted.

_____ 6. Airway partially obstructed by secretions. Plan to use bulb syringe for suctioning.

115. After being awake for 60 minutes after birth, a neonate falls asleep. Which responses should a nurse determine are normal when the neonate is in this sleep phase after birth? **Select all that apply.**

1. Displays decreased muscle activity.
2. Startles easily to external stimuli.
3. Perspiration present on the neonate's skin.
4. Respiratory rate 45 breaths per minute.
5. Heart rate 120 beats per minute.

114. ANSWER: 2, 5, 6, 1, 3, 4.
The nurse should first document the initial observations: *Small amount of clear thick mucus draining from both nares.* Next, the nurse should assess the respiratory status of the infant to determine whether the suctioning will be tolerated: *Respirations 62 per minute, breathing without difficulty, and no retractions noted.* Next, the nurse should analyze the data and plan an intervention: *Airway partially obstructed by secretions. Plan to use bulb syringe for suctioning.* The nurse should then state the procedure performed: *Both nares suctioned with bulb syringe* and then the results: *Suctioning produced small amount of clear thick mucus.* Finally, the nurse should evaluate how the procedure was tolerated and the effectiveness of the intervention: *Procedure tolerated and respirations returned to normal rate, suctioning effective to clear the secretions.*

TEST-TAKING TIP: Use the nursing process steps of assessment, analysis, planning, implementation, and evaluation to place the statements in the correct order.

Content Area: Childbearing Families; **Category of Health Alteration:** Neonatal and High Risk Neonatal Management; **Integrated Processes:** Communication and Documentation; **Client Need:** Physiological Integrity/Reduction of Risk Potential/ Changes or Abnormalities in Vital Signs; **Cognitive Level:** Analysis; **References:** Potter, P., & Perry, A. (2009), pp. 349–358; Ward, S., & Hisley, S. (2009), p. 565.

115. ANSWER: 1, 4, 5.
During the sleep phase the infant displays decreased muscle activity and is resting quietly recovering from the stress of birth. The respiratory rate is within the normal range of 30–60 breaths per minute. The heart rate is within the normal range of 120–160 beats per minute. When in the sleep phase, a neonate is difficult to awaken. The sweat glands are not fully functional until after the first month of life.

TEST-TAKING TIP: Visualize a neonate during the initial sleep phase after birth to answer this question.

Content Area: Childbearing Families; **Category of Health Alteration:** Neonatal and High Risk Neonatal Management; **Integrated Processes:** Nursing Process Evaluation; **Client Need:** Health Promotion and Maintenance/Ante/Intra/Postpartum and Newborn Care; **Cognitive Level:** Application; **Reference:** Ward, S., & Hisley, S. (2009), pp. 549, 558, 571.

116. A nurse completes a newborn assessment. After inspecting the newborn's hand illustrated, which conclusion by the nurse is correct?

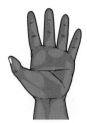

1. The newborn's palmar crease is a normal finding.
2. The newborn definitely has Down's syndrome.
3. The newborn has a simian crease, which may be insignificant.
4. The newborn has syndactyly, which may be a significant finding.

117. A nurse is caring for a small-for-gestational-age (SGA) newborn. Which interventions should the nurse plan to prevent heat loss? **Select all that apply.**

1. Lay the newborn on a heating pad.
2. Wrap the newborn in blankets that were warmed in a warmer.
3. Have the mother hold the infant skin-to-skin next to the mother's chest.
4. Apply a stockinette head covering.
5. Place the newborn under a radiant warmer if the newborn's axillary temperature is 97.7°F (36.5°C).

116. ANSWER: 3.
A simian crease is a single, straight crease appearing in the middle of the palm on one or both hands. When unaccompanied by other abnormal findings, the simian crease is insignificant. The hands of a normal neonate usually contain three or four curved palmar creases. A simian crease, when detected along with other symptoms, may be associated with Down's syndrome or other syndromes. Syndactyly is a webbing of the skin between the digits. No webbing is present.

TEST-TAKING TIP: The palm shows a simian crease. Use this information to narrow the options to 2 and 3. Of these options, consider that little information is provided in the question to draw a definite conclusion.

Content Area: Childbearing Families; **Category of Health Alteration:** Neonatal and High Risk Neonatal Management; **Integrated Processes:** Nursing Process Analysis; **Client Need:** Health Promotion and Maintenance/Ante/Intra/Postpartum and Newborn Care; **Cognitive Level:** Analysis; **Reference:** Ward, S., & Hisley, S. (2009), pp. 588–589.

117. ANSWER: 2, 3, 4.
Wrapping the newborn in blankets warmed in a warmer is an effective, albeit temporary, heat source. Kangaroo care (skin-to-skin holding of an infant dressed only in a diaper) is an effective method for maintaining a newborn's temperature. A stockinette hat prevents heat loss through the head. A heating pad can cause burn injuries. A normal axillary temperature is 97.7°F–99.5°F (36.5°C–37.5°C); a radiant warmer is used if the temperature is below normal or if the newborn cannot maintain an adequate temperature.

TEST-TAKING TIP: Eliminate any option that injures the newborn or is unnecessary to maintain the newborn's body temperature.

Content Area: Childbearing Families; **Category of Health Alteration:** Neonatal and High Risk Neonatal Management; **Integrated Processes:** Caring; Nursing Process Planning; **Client Need:** Health Promotion and Maintenance/Ante/Intra/Postpartum and Newborn Care; **Cognitive Level:** Application; **Reference:** Ward, S., & Hisley, S. (2009), pp. 606–607.

Test 12: Childbearing Families: Pharmacological and Parenteral Therapies

118. A pregnant client who is prescribed supplemental vitamin D during pregnancy asks the nurse why vitamin D is so important. Which responses by the nurse are correct? **Select all that apply.**

1. "Almost 50% of pregnant women lack sufficient vitamin D levels during late pregnancy."
2. "A low level of vitamin D is associated with reduced bone-mineral accumulation during your child's growing years."
3. "A low level of vitamin D may predispose you to premature rupture of your membranes."
4. "A low level of vitamin D causes a breakdown of cervical collagen, prompting early cervical dilation."
5. "Vitamin D supplements taken during pregnancy may reduce the risk for osteoporosis-related fractures in your offspring."

119. Which agents if prescribed by a health care provider (HCP) to treat a client with hyperemesis gravidarum should a nurse question? **Select all that apply.**

1. Pyridoxine (vitamin B$_6$) 50 mg oral daily
2. Promethazine (Phenergan) 12.5 mg IV q4h
3. Dimenhydrinate (Dramamine) 50 mg oral q4–6 h prn
4. Metoclopramide (Reglan) 100 mg IM q8h
5. Ginger capsule 1 g oral daily
6. Prochlorperazine (Compazine) 30 mg oral daily

118. ANSWER: 1, 2, 5.

Research has shown that vitamin D levels during late pregnancy were insufficient in 31% and deficient in 18% of pregnant women. A low level of vitamin D is associated with an offspring's reduced bone-mineral accumulation at age 9 years and supplements taken during pregnancy may reduce their risk for osteoporosis-related fractures. A low level of vitamin C (not D) predisposes a woman to premature rupture of the membranes. The lack of vitamin C (not D) increases the rate of cervical collagen degradation. With decreased collagen, the cervix ripens more easily, prompting effacement and dilation.

TEST-TAKING TIP: Recall that vitamin D is essential for the absorption of calcium. Use this information to select options related to the bones. Eliminate options not related to bone growth.

Content Area: Childbearing Families; **Category of Health Alteration:** Pharmacological and Parenteral Therapies; **Integrated Processes:** Teaching and Learning; **Client Need:** Physiological Integrity/Pharmacological and Parenteral Therapies/Expected Actions or Outcomes; **Cognitive Level:** Application; **Reference:** Ward, S., & Hisley, S. (2009), pp. 234, 257; **EBP Reference:** Javaid, M.K., Crozier, S., Harvey, N., Dennison, E., Arden, N., Godfrey, K., & Cooper, C. (2006). Maternal vitamin D status during pregnancy and childhood bone mass at age 9 years: A longitudinal study. *The Lancet, 367,* 36–43.

119. ANSWER: 4, 6.

The dose of metoclopramide is 10 times the usual dose; it should be 10 mg and not 100 mg. Prochlorperazine is a pregnancy category C drug indicating that its safety has not been established for use during pregnancy. Pyridoxine, promethazine, dimenhydrinate, and ginger have antiemetic effects and are medications for treating nausea and vomiting of pregnancy. The dose, route, and frequency of these medications are within the recommended ranges.

TEST-TAKING TIP: All agents listed are used to treat nausea and vomiting. Eliminate any option that exceeds the recommended dosage range or is a pregnancy category C drug.

Content Area: Childbearing Families; **Category of Health Alteration:** Pharmacological and Parenteral Therapies; **Integrated Processes:** Communication and Documentation; **Client Need:** Physiological Integrity/Pharmacological and Parenteral Therapies/Medication Administration; **Cognitive Level:** Analysis; **References:** Deglin, J., & Vallerand, A. (2011), p. 847; Ward, S., & Hisley, S. (2009), p. 297.

120. A nurse reviews the serum laboratory report for a client who developed a deep vein thrombosis and is to receive warfarin (Coumadin) 5 mg orally now. Based on the results of the serum laboratory report, which action should be taken by the nurse?

Serum Laboratory Report	Client Values
PT (9.2–11.9 sec)	12.8 sec
INR (0.9–1.1 sec)	1.9 sec
APTT (24–33 sec)	36 sec
Hgb (11.1–15.5 g/dL)	11 g/dL
Hct (38–44%)	33%
Platelets (PLT 150,000–400,000/mm³)	120,000/mm³

1. Notify the health care provider (HCP) to question the dose.
2. Administer the warfarin as prescribed.
3. Reduce the dose of warfarin to 2.5 mg.
4. Reschedule warfarin to be given later in the day.

121. A nurse is assisting with the administration of spinal anesthesia in preparation for a cesarean birth. The nurse gathers equipment, explains the procedure to the client, and performs hand hygiene. Place the nurse's remaining steps in the correct numerical order (1–6).

_____ 1. Document the procedure, client's vital signs, and fetal heart rate (FHR).

_____ 2. Assist the client to a sitting position with the client's head bowed and the back arched.

_____ 3. Assist the client to lie down on her back.

_____ 4. After medication administration and repositioning, evaluate vital signs and fetal FHR.

_____ 5. Stand at the front of the client and support the client's shoulders.

_____ 6. Place a pillow under the client's head and a wedge under her right hip.

120. ANSWER: 2.
The dosing of warfarin is adjusted based on the international normalized ratio (INR) results. A normal therapeutic INR is 2.0–3.5. The client's INR has not yet reached therapeutic levels. It is unnecessary to notify the HCP; the dose is within the recommended range of 2.5 to 10 mg daily. The nurse should not reduce a dose without first consulting the HCP. A "now" medication is to be given within 30 to 60 minutes of receiving the order.

TEST-TAKING TIP: Consider that warfarin inhibits the hepatic synthesis of coagulation factors to prevent clotting. Prothrombin time (PT) and INR are used to evaluate the effectiveness of warfarin as an anticoagulant. Focus on these two values when selecting an option.

Content Area: Childbearing Families; **Category of Health Alteration:** Pharmacological and Parenteral Therapies; **Integrated Processes:** Nursing Process Analysis; **Client Need:** Physiological Integrity/Pharmacological and Parenteral Therapies/Expected Actions or Outcomes; **Cognitive Level:** Analysis; **Reference:** Ward, S., & Hisley, S. (2009), pp. 199, 529.

121. ANSWER: 2, 5, 3, 6, 4, 1.
First, assist the client to a sitting position with the client's head bowed and her back arched. Next, stand at the front of the client and support the client's shoulders. This will prevent the client from falling. After the anesthesia has been delivered, assist the client to lie down on her back. Then place a pillow under the client's head and a wedge under her right hip. The woman's vital signs are assessed every 1–2 minutes for 10 minutes, then every 5–10 minutes. Fetal heart rate (FHR) is continuously monitored with electronic monitoring and should be evaluated after medication administration and repositioning. Finally, document the procedure, client's vital signs, and FHR in the client's chart.

TEST-TAKING TIP: Visualize assisting with a spinal anesthesia before placing actions in the correct sequence. The client is usually in a sitting position when receiving spinal anesthesia.

Content Area: Childbearing Families; **Category of Health Alteration:** Pharmacological and Parenteral Therapies; **Integrated Processes:** Nursing Process Implementation; **Client Need:** Physiological Integrity/Pharmacological and Parenteral Therapies/Pharmacological Pain Management; **Cognitive Level:** Application; **Reference:** Ward, S., & Hisley, S. (2009), p. 418.

122. Which findings during a nurse's assessment of a pregnant client should prompt the nurse to lower the dose or discontinue an oxytocin (Pitocin) infusion? **Select all that apply.**

1. Uterine contractions lasting greater than 90 seconds, and occur more frequently than every 2 minutes
2. Repeated late decelerations
3. Uterine resting tone 10 mm Hg
4. Fetal heart rate (FHR) baseline 140 beats per minute (bpm)
5. Vaginal bleeding, tachycardia, and hypotension

123. A client is prescribed a maintenance dose of magnesium sulfate 2 g/hr intravenously for preterm labor. Magnesium sulfate is supplied in a solution of 40 g in 1,000 mL of lactated Ringer's solution. At how many milliliters (mL) per hour should the nurse plan to set the infusion pump to deliver the medication?

_____ mL (Record your answer as a whole number.)

122. ANSWER: 1, 2, 5.
Uterine contractions lasting greater than 90 seconds and occurring more frequently than every 2 minutes and fetal heart rate decelerations are signs of uterine hyperstimulation. Research suggests there is a significant increase in the number of women requiring epidural analgesia with the use of oxytocin. Vaginal bleeding, tachycardia, and hypotension could indicate uterine rupture from overstimulation of the uterus. Uterine resting tone greater than 20 mm Hg (not 10) and a FHR baseline of less than 100 or greater than 160 bpm are other signs of uterine hyperstimulation. A FHR baseline of 140 bpm is within the normal range.

TEST-TAKING TIP: Eliminate options with normal findings (3 and 4).

Content Area: Childbearing Families; **Category of Health Alteration:** Pharmacological and Parenteral Therapies; **Integrated Processes:** Nursing Process Evaluation; **Client Need:** Physiological Integrity/Pharmacological and Parenteral Therapies/Adverse Effects/Contraindications/Interactions; **Cognitive Level:** Analysis; **Reference:** Word, S., & Hisley, S. (2009), pp. 435–436; **EBP Reference:** Alfirevic, Z., Kelly, A.J., & Dowswell, T. (2009). Intravenous oxytocin alone for cervical ripening and induction of labour. *Cochrane Database of Systematic Reviews* 2009, Issue 4. Art. No.: CD003246. DOI: 10.1002/14651858. CD003246.pub2. Retrieved from http://www.cochrane.org/reviews/en/ab003246.html

123. ANSWER: 50
Use a proportion formula to determine the amount of solution in milliliters for 2 g of medication. Multiply the outside values and then inside values and solve for *X*.

40 g : 1,000 mL :: 2 g : *X* mL

40 *X* = 2,000

X = 50

TEST-TAKING TIP: The total amount of medication and solution is 40 g in 1,000 mL. To administer 2 g/hr, you need to determine the amount of solution in milliliters for 2 g of medication.

Content Area: Childbearing Families; **Category of Health Alteration:** Pharmacological and Parenteral Therapies; **Integrated Processes:** Nursing Process Planning; **Client Need:** Physiological Integrity/Pharmacological and Parenteral Therapies/Dosage Calculation; **Cognitive Level:** Application; **References:** Pickar, G., & Abernethy, A. (2008), p. 46; Ward, S., & Hisley, S. (2009), p. 309.

Tab 4   **Physiological Integrity** | Adult
          Health

Test 13: Adult Health: Developmental Needs

124. A 45-year-old client calls a clinic for the third time in a month with concerns of indigestion and requests a prescription to "take care of her indigestion." She refuses an x-ray examination because she "can't fit it into her busy work schedule." She owns her own successful consulting business. Her husband recently quit his job and is staying home to monitor the activities of their 14-year-old daughter, who has been skipping school. Based on this information, which conclusions by the nurse are correct concerning the client's psychosocial developmental characteristics and tasks associated with middle-aged adulthood? **Select all that apply.**

1. The client has established an economic standard of living.
2. The client lacks leisure-time activities.
3. The client is unable to balance the needs of multiple demands without untoward effects.
4. The client is in the stagnation phase of Erikson's stages of development.
5. The client is assisting her daughter to become a responsible and happy adult.

125. A clinic nurse is reviewing the physical assessment findings of a 52-year-old female. Which set of findings should the nurse conclude are normal age-related changes for this client?

Physical Findings

1.	Eyes	Reduced peripheral vision, drooping of the upper lids
2.	Breasts	Orange-peel appearance, small nodules around areola
3.	Musculoskeletal System	Decreased strength against resistance, lordosis
4.	Integument	Wrinkling of the skin, jaundice

124. ANSWER: 1, 2, 3.

Characteristics of middle-age development include establishing and maintaining an economic standard of living (her consulting business has been successful), developing adult leisure-time activities (she lacks time for these), and balancing the needs of multiple demands (her indigestion and comments suggest that she is unable to balance these needs without untoward effects). She is in the generativity phase of Erikson's stages of development (not stagnation). The spouse is monitoring the daughter's activities.

TEST-TAKING TIP: Read each option carefully, noting these key words in the options: "has established," "lacks," "unable," "stagnation," and "assisting." Then, reread the situation. Erikson's stage of development for middle adulthood is generativity versus stagnation.

Content Area: Adult Health; **Category of Health Alteration:** Developmental Needs; **Integrated Processes:** Nursing Process Analysis; **Client Need:** Health Promotion and Maintenance/Health and Wellness; **Cognitive Level:** Analysis; **Reference:** Berman, A., Snyder, S., Kozier, B., & Erb, G. (2008), pp. 398–399.

125. ANSWER: 1.

Reduced peripheral vision, ptosis, asymmetric position of the light reflex, and redness or crusting around the eyelids are normal age-related changes in the middle-aged adult. A nodule (elevated, palpable, solid mass), lordosis (curvature of the spine), and jaundiced skin (yellow pigmentation) are not normal age-related changes.

TEST-TAKING TIP: Examine each option carefully to identify an abnormal finding in three of the four options.

Content Area: Adult Health; **Category of Health Alteration:** Developmental Needs; **Integrated Processes:** Nursing Process Evaluation; **Client Need:** Health Promotion and Maintenance/Health and Wellness; **Cognitive Level:** Application; **Reference:** Potter, P., & Perry, A. (2009), pp. 184–185.

126. A nurse is caring for a group of clients with various needs. In which order should the nurse address clients' needs? Place the clients in the numerical order (1–5) in which their needs should be addressed.

_____ 1. A 40-year-old client who refuses to participate in self-care because her "body looks so terrible" after having one breast removed due to cancer

_____ 2. A 35-year-old client who has an oxygen saturation level of 77%

_____ 3. A 55-year-old client who just learned that her husband died in the same car accident that resulted in her hospitalization

_____ 4. A 53-year-old client who wants to bring his home computer to do some work and check for feedback from his recently published work that he feels has been a success

_____ 5. A 76-year-old client who is threatening to leave the hospital because of poor care

127. Which statements made by a 48-year-old female during a clinic visit **best** reflect the normal characteristics and developmental tasks associated with middle adulthood? **Select all that apply.**

1. "I have been staying active by joining a golf league."
2. "I am so tired in the mornings that I am less motivated to go to work now than when I was younger."
3. "My husband and I will be caring for our grandson while my son and his wife look at a new home they want to purchase."
4. "I have been volunteering for the clothing drive once a month through the Epilepsy Foundation."
5. "My body has gotten so out of shape that I don't like to go out much anymore."

126. ANSWER: 2, 5, 3, 1, 4.
Using Maslow's Hierarchy of Needs theory as a guide, the 35-year-old client should be seen first because the client has a basic physiological need for oxygen. Next, the nurse should attend to the 76-year-old client who is threatening to leave the hospital because the client has a physical safety need. Third, the nurse should attend to the 55-year-old client because she is grieving and has a need for psychological safety and love and belonging. The 40-year-old client has a self-esteem need and should be attended to next. Finally, the nurse should attend to the 53-year-old client who has reached the point of self-actualization.

TEST-TAKING TIP: Use Maslow's Hierarchy of Needs theory to place the options in the correct sequence.

Content Area: Adult Health; **Category of Health Alteration:** Developmental Needs; **Integrated Processes:** Nursing Process Planning; **Client Need:** Safe and Effective Care Environment/Management of Care/Establishing Priorities; **Cognitive Level:** Analysis; **Reference:** Potter, P., & Perry, A. (2009), pp. 71–72.

127. ANSWER: 1, 3, 4.
Significant characteristics and developmental tasks of middle adulthood include developing adult leisure-time activities, assisting children to become responsible adults, and achieving adult civic and social responsibility. Responses in options 2 and 5 suggest that the client has not adjusted to the physiological changes associated with middle age.

TEST-TAKING TIP: The key word is "normal." Eliminate options that include negativity.

Content Area: Adult Health; **Category of Health Alteration:** Developmental Needs; **Integrated Processes:** Nursing Process Assessment; **Client Need:** Health Promotion and Maintenance/Health and Wellness; **Cognitive Level:** Application; **Reference:** Berman, A., Snyder, S., Kozier, B., & Erb, G. (2008), pp. 351–355.

Test 14: Adult Health: Older Client Needs

128. A nurse is teaching nursing assistants newly hired to work in a long-term care facility. Which information regarding the residents' skin care should the nurse emphasize? **Select all that apply.**

1. Avoid skin products that contain alcohol.
2. Apply perfumed skin lotions after the resident's bath when the skin is still moist.
3. Apply sunscreen lotions with a sun protection factor (SPF) of 8 when residents are in the sun.
4. Send soiled clothing to the laundry where strong detergents can be used to remove food stains.
5. Use soft washcloths and towels when bathing the residents.

129. An 85-year-old female client is brought to the emergency department by her son who found his mother lying on the floor. She is alert, but confused. The client is taking warfarin (Coumadin) for chronic atrial fibrillation and amiodarone (Cordarone). Which actions should be taken by a nurse after reviewing the client's serum laboratory report? **Select all that apply.**

1. Assess the client for signs of bleeding.
2. Insert a urinary drainage catheter.
3. Monitor for a decrease in level of consciousness (LOC).
4. Notify the health care provider (HCP) of the results.
5. Anticipate receiving an order for vitamin K.
6. Obtain a 12-lead electrocardiogram (ECG).

Serum Laboratory Value	Client Value
CK-MB (0–16 mcg/L)	33 mcg/L
Troponin (0.0–0.4 ng/mL)	42 ng/mL
BUN (7–23 mg/dL)	30 mg/dL
SCr (0.4–1.4 mg/dL)	3.8 mg/dL
PT (11–13 sec)	32 seconds
INR (0.9–1.1 sec)	5

128. ANSWER: 1, 5.
Age-related skin changes of the elderly include dry and fragile skin. **Alcohol is drying to the skin and should be avoided. Using soft washcloths and towels will prevent skin injury.** Perfume-free skin lotions should be used because perfumed lotions increase skin irritation. Sunscreen should have an SPF of 15 or greater to protect against sunburn. Strong laundry detergents should be avoided because of skin irritation and the risk of skin breakdown.

TEST-TAKING TIP: If unsure, note the key word "avoid" in option 1, which is an opposite action as compared to most other options. Of the other options, select an option that would avoid tissue injury.

Content Area: Adult Health; **Category of Health Alteration:** Older Client Needs; **Integrated Processes:** Teaching and Learning; **Client Need:** Health Promotion and Maintenance/Aging Process; **Cognitive Level:** Application; **Reference:** Berman, A., Snyder, S., Kozier, B., & Erb, G. (2008), p. 411.

129. ANSWER: 1, 3, 4, 5, 6.
The PT (prothrombin time) and international normalized ratio (INR) are excessively elevated; the client is at a high risk for bleeding. A change in LOC could suggest a hemorrhagic stroke. The HCP should be notified of the findings immediately. Vitamin K will counteract the anticoagulant effects of warfarin. The cardiac enzymes are also elevated (CK-MB and troponin), indicating a myocardial infarction (MI). A 12-lead ECG is needed to evaluate the location of the MI. Although the serum creatinine (SCr) and blood urea nitrogen (BUN) are elevated, the client is alert and a urinary catheter is unnecessary and could cause further trauma and bleeding.

TEST-TAKING TIP: Note that all laboratory values are abnormal. CK-MB and troponin are cardiac enzymes, BUN and SCr are tests of renal function, and PT and INR are tests for coagulation. Use this information to select the correct options.

Content Area: Adult Health; **Category of Health Alteration:** Older Client Needs; **Integrated Processes:** Nursing Process Implementation; **Client Need:** Physiological Integrity/Reduction of Risk Potential/Laboratory Values; **Cognitive Level:** Analysis; **Reference:** Mauk, K. (2010), pp. 271–272.

130. A home health nurse suspects elder mistreatment of a 93-year-old client by a live-in caregiver. Which findings supported the nurse's conclusion? **Select all that apply.**

1. Client has urine burns.
2. Client has wrist bruises.
3. Client states there have been some unexplained financial expenditures.
4. Client is more talkative than during previous home visits.
5. Smell of alcohol noted on live-in caregiver's breath.

131. A nurse completed teaching for a client diagnosed with glaucoma. Which statements made by the client indicates that the teaching was effective? **Select all that apply.**

1. "Medical follow-up and my eye medication will be required for the rest of my life."
2. "I need to continue my eye drops for as long as prescribed, even in the absence of symptoms."
3. "I plan to discourage my daughter's constant rearranging of my furniture."
4. "Wearing eye patches when I go to bed will prevent morning glare on waking."
5. "My MedicAlert bracelet identifies that I have glaucoma and lists the eye drops prescribed."
6. "It is safe for me to drive immediately after instilling my eyedrops."

130. ANSWER: 1, 2, 3, 5.

Urine burns suggest caregiver neglect. Wrist bruises suggest physical abuse. Unexplained financial expenditures suggest financial exploitation. Substance abuse is an abuser characteristic. A more withdrawn client, rather than a more talkative one suggests psychological or emotional abuse.

TEST-TAKING TIP: Apply knowledge of elder mistreatment, which is an umbrella term for abuse, exploitation, and neglect.

Content Area: Adult Health; **Category of Health Alteration:** Older Client Needs; **Integrated Processes:** Nursing Process Analysis; **Client Need:** Psychosocial Integrity/ Abuse/Neglect; **Cognitive Level:** Analysis; **Reference:** Townsend, M. (2011), pp. 684–686; **EBP Reference:** Fulmer, T. (2008). Elder Mistreatment and Abuse Assessment. *The Hartford Institute for Geriatric Nursing: Best Practices to Nursing Care of Adult Health,* Issue 15. Retrieved from www.hartfordign.org/publications/trythis/issue15.pdf

131. ANSWER: 1, 2, 3, 5.

Glaucoma is a chronic illness necessitating continued medical supervision and medication to allay problems as the disease progresses. The client should continue the eye drops, even after the blurred vision decreases. Medications that dilate the pupil increase intraocular pressure. The client should also notify health care providers about taking eye drops for glaucoma treatment and check with a pharmacist before taking any over-the-counter drugs. It is best to leave furniture the way the client is used to it being arranged for client safety. Clients are advised to wear a MedicAlert® bracelet or carry a medical alert card to inform medical personnel in emergency situations. Wearing an eye patch further limits the client's vision causing safety concerns. Driving is avoided for 1–2 hours after administering eyedrops for treating glaucoma.

TEST-TAKING TIP: Knowledge of glaucoma and miotics is needed to select the answers. Use the "o" as a memory cue in mi**o**tics to remember that mi**o**tics c**o**nstrict the pupil.

Content Area: Adult Health; **Category of Health Alteration:** Older Client Needs; **Integrated Processes:** Nursing Process Evaluation; **Client Need:** Health Promotion and Maintenance/Self-care; **Cognitive Level:** Application; **References:** Ignatavicius, D., & Workman, M. (2010), pp. 1095–1098; Wilson, B., Shannon, M., Shields, K., & Stang, C. (2008), pp. 1216–1218.

132. A nurse observes the following findings during an assessment of a 68-year-old client. Which finding should the nurse conclude is a normal age-related change to the client's skin?

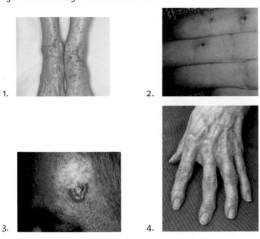

1.

2.

3.

4.

133. A home health nurse is assessing family functioning of a client who has human immunodeficiency virus (HIV). Which questions should the nurse ask the client? **Select all that apply.**

1. "How are decisions made in the family?"
2. "What types of activities does the family engage in as a group?"
3. "How many brothers and sisters do you have?"
4. "What are important family beliefs and how does each member carry out the beliefs?"
5. "Do you consider the relationships between and among family members to be healthy and supportive?"

132. ANSWER: 4.
Skin changes include loss of skin elasticity, reduced skin thickness, and loss of subcutaneous fat. The other skin changes are abnormal. Option 1 shows petechiae, the tiny red spots associated with microembolism. Option 2 shows Osler's nodes (small, painless nodes on fingers and toes) from cardiac emboli. Option 3 shows squamous cell carcinoma.

TEST-TAKING TIP: Focus just on the client's skin to select the correct option. Avoid reading into the question.

Content Area: Adult Health; **Category of Health Alteration:** Older Client Needs; **Integrated Processes:** Nursing Process Assessment; **Client Need:** Health Promotion and Maintenance/Aging Process; **Cognitive Level:** Application; **Reference:** Berman, A., Snyder, S., Kozier, B., & Erb, G. (2008), pp. 412–413.

133. ANSWER: 1, 2, 4, 5.
The nurse should ask questions to elicit the various aspects of family functioning. Question 1 assesses family cognition and perception. Question 2 assesses family activity and exercise. Question 4 assesses family beliefs and values. Question 5 assesses family roles and relationships. Asking the numbers of brothers and sisters does not assess family functioning.

TEST-TAKING TIP: Asking a question that expects a numerical response would not provide information about family function. Eliminate option 3.

Content Area: Adult Health; **Category of Health Alteration:** Older Client Needs; **Integrated Processes:** Nursing Process Assessment; **Client Need:** Health Promotion and Maintenance/Developmental Stages and Transitions; **Cognitive Level:** Application; **Reference:** Craven, R., & Hirnle, C. (2009), p. 300; **EBP Reference:** Van Horn, E. (2007, May/Jun). Promotion of family integrity in the acute care setting: a review of the literature. *Dimensions of Critical Care Nursing, 26*(3), pp. 101–107.

Test 15: Adult Health: Cardiac Management

134. A client at high risk for coronary artery disease (CAD) is receiving instructions for a 2,000-Kcalorie heart-healthy diet. Which statements are likely to be made by a nurse during the teaching session? **Select all that apply.**

1. Limit your intake of foods that are high in omega-3 fatty acids.
2. Keep colorful foods such as carrots, grapes, blueberries, and melon in the refrigerator.
3. Use lean ground turkey instead of ground beef.
4. Limit meat, fish, and poultry servings to a maximum of 3 ounces per day.
5. Add unsalted nuts to meals to increase monounsaturated fat intake.
6. Avoid margarines with added plant sterols, which increase LDL cholesterol levels.

135. A nurse is preparing discharge instructions for a client who recently had a cardiac catheterization through the femoral artery. Which instructions should be essential elements of the nurse's discharge plan? **Select all that apply.**

1. Remove the pressure dressing the day after the catheterization.
2. Keep the puncture site covered for several days.
3. Soak in the bathtub to remove the antiseptic dye.
4. Observe the site for redness, swelling, drainage, and bruising.
5. Avoid strenuous exercise for the next few days.
6. Call the health care provider (HCP) if a lump is palpated or swelling is noted in the groin.

134. ANSWER: 2, 3, 5.
A healthy 2000-Kcalorie diet includes eating 2½ cups of vegetables and two fruits daily. Keeping colorful foods in the refrigerator makes it easier to choose a healthy food when the urge for a snack arises. Poultry products are lower in fat than beef products. Adding unsalted nuts to meals increases monounsaturated fat intake and can make meals more appetizing. Omega-3 fatty acids in fatty fish may reduce CAD risk because fish are low in saturated fat. Also, the omega-3 fatty acids have been shown to suppress the inflammatory response, reduce blood clotting, stabilize heart rhythm, and lower triglyceride levels in people who have had a heart attack. Meat, fish, and poultry servings should be limited to 5½ ounces daily. Tub margarines with added plant sterols help to lower LDL cholesterol levels.

TEST-TAKING TIP: Look for key words in each of the options that would make the option either right or wrong for a 2,000-Kcalorie diet.

Content Area: Adult Health; **Category of Health Alteration:** Cardiac Management; **Integrated Processes:** Teaching and Learning; **Client Need:** Physiological Integrity/ Basic Care and Comfort/Nutrition and Oral Hydration; **Cognitive Level:** Application; **Reference:** Lutz, C., & Przytulski, K. (2011), pp. 379–387.

135. ANSWER: 1, 2, 4, 5, 6.
A pressure dressing reduces the risk of arterial bleeding. Leaving the pressure dressing on too long can impair circulation. Usually, only a small bandage is required after the pressure dressing is removed. This should be changed daily. The site should be observed for signs of infection. Avoiding strenuous activity decreases the risk of disrupting the clot and bleeding from the puncture site. A developing hematoma can be palpated in the groin and can be an early sign of a leaking vessel. A tub bath should be avoided until the puncture site heals to decrease the risk of infection.

TEST-TAKING TIP: Recall that a vessel is catheterized during the procedure. Focus on teaching to promote healing, preventing infection, preventing bleeding and other complications, and when to notify the HCP.

Content Area: Adult Health; **Category of Health Alteration:** Cardiac Management; **Integrated Processes:** Nursing Process Planning; **Client Need:** Physiological Integrity/Reduction of Risk Potential/Potential for Complications of Diagnostic Tests/Treatments/Procedures; **Cognitive Level:** Analysis; **Reference:** Smeltzer, S., Bare, B., Hinkle, J., & Cheever, K. (2010), pp. 713–715.

136. A nurse responds to a client's ECG monitor alarm. Which should be the nurse's interpretation for the following electrocardiogram (ECG) rhythm?

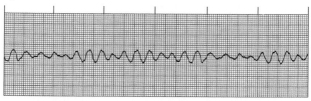

1. Atrial flutter
2. Atrial fibrillation
3. Ventricular fibrillation
4. Ventricular tachycardia

137. A nurse is reviewing the care plan of a client who has a nursing diagnosis of *Ineffective cardiac tissue perfusion related to reduced coronary blood flow following an uncomplicated myocardial infarction (MI)*. Which observations should prompt a nurse to conclude that expected outcomes for this nursing diagnosis have been met? **Select all that apply.**

1. Oxygen administered at 2 liters per nasal cannula
2. Heart rate reduced from 110 beats per minute (bpm) to 70 bpm after treatment with metoprolol (Lopressor)
3. ECG shows sinus rhythm with no ST segment elevation
4. Reports absence of chest pain and dyspnea
5. S_1, S_2, and S_3 heart sounds present

136. ANSWER: 3.
In ventricular fibrillation, the HR is not measurable, the rhythm is irregular and chaotic, the P wave is not visible, and the PR interval and QRS complex are not measurable. In atrial flutter, the atrial rate is measurable between 250 to 350 beats per minute (bpm), the rhythm can be regular or irregular, the P waves are discernible, the PR interval is variable and not measurable, and the QRS complex is usually normal. In atrial fibrillation, the atrial rate is not measurable, the ventricular rate is measurable, the rhythm is irregular, the P waves are fibrillatory, the PR interval is not measurable, and the QRS complex is usually normal. In ventricular tachycardia, the ventricular rate is measurable between 150 to 250 bpm, the rhythm is regular or irregular, P waves are usually buried in the QRS complex, the PR interval is not measurable, and the QRS complex has a distorted appearance with a duration exceeding 0.12 second.

TEST-TAKING TIP: Use the steps in interpreting an ECG rhythm to select the correct option. Note the fibrillatory waves and eliminate options 1 and 4. Eliminate option 2 because the rhythm strip shows unmeasurable QRS complexes.

Content Area: Adult Health; **Category of Health Alteration:** Cardiac Management; **Integrated Processes:** Nursing Process Analysis; **Client Need:** Physiological Integrity/Physiological Adaptation/Hemodynamics; **Cognitive Level:** Analysis; **Reference:** Ignatavicius, D., & Workman, M. (2010), pp. 748–749.

137. ANSWER: 2, 3, 4.
A beta-blocker is a first-line medication given to preserve myocardial tissue. It blocks the stimulation of beta$_1$-adrenergic receptors, thus decreasing blood pressure and heart rate. Sinus rhythm without ST segment elevation indicates the absence of ischemia and injury. The absence of chest pain indicates the heart is adequately perfused. The administration of oxygen is an intervention and not an outcome. The presence of a S_3 heart sound indicates decreased left ventricular compliance associated with the MI.

TEST-TAKING TIP: Eliminate any options that are interventions. Then eliminate abnormal assessment findings. Select only normal findings that indicate that the reduced coronary blood flow has been resolved.

Content Area: Adult Health; **Category of Health Alteration:** Cardiac Management; **Integrated Processes:** Nursing Process Analysis; **Client Need:** Safe and Effective Care Environment/Management of Care/Continuity of Care; **Cognitive Level:** Analysis; **Reference:** Smeltzer, S., Bare, B., Hinkle, J., & Cheever, K. (2010), p. 775.

138. A client admitted with left ventricular heart failure has sudden onset breathlessness and a sense of suffocation while sitting in a chair. The client's pulse is weak and rapid, and neck veins are distended. Which actions should be taken by a nurse? **Select all that apply.**

1. Assist the client to bed and place the bed in a flat position.
2. Initiate oxygen via a facemask.
3. Administer morphine sulfate 4 mg intravenously (IV).
4. Prepare to administer furosemide (Lasix) IV.
5. Prepare to administer cyclophosphamide (Cytoxan) IV.

139. A client who has systolic heart failure is to receive enalapril (Enalaprilat) 0.625 mg IV. The nurse obtains the medication from the automated dispensing system, which has the label illustrated. How many milliliters (mL) of medication should the nurse prepare for the correct dose?

_____ mL (Record your answer to the nearest tenth.)

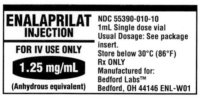

ENALAPRILAT
INJECTION
FOR IV USE ONLY
1.25 mg/mL
(Anhydrous equivalent)

NDC 55390-010-10
1mL Single dose vial
Usual Dosage: See package insert.
Store below 30°C (86°F)
Rx ONLY
Manufactured for:
Bedford Labs™
Bedford, OH 44146 ENL-W01

138. ANSWER: 2, 3, 4.
A facemask is used initially for oxygen therapy in pulmonary edema to relieve hypoxemia and dyspnea. Morphine will reduce peripheral resistance and venous return so that blood can be redistributed from the pulmonary circulation to other body systems. Furosemide promotes the excretion of sodium and water; it also causes vasodilation and pooling of blood in peripheral blood vessels, which reduces the amount of blood returning to the heart. The client should be positioned upright, preferably with the legs dangling over the side of the bed, to reduce venous return to the heart. Cyclophosphamide is an immunosuppressant and antineoplastic medication and would be an inappropriate medication in treating pulmonary edema.

TEST-TAKING TIP: The focus of the question is on interventions for treating pulmonary edema. Eliminate actions that will further compromise the airway and administering an immunosuppressant medication.

Content Area: Adult Health; **Category of Health Alteration:** Cardiac Management; **Integrated Processes:** Nursing Process Implementation; **Client Need:** Physiological Integrity/Physiological Adaptation/Medical Emergencies; **Cognitive Level:** Analysis; **References:** Deglin, J., & Vallerand, A. (2011), pp. 384, 620; Smeltzer, S., Bare, B., Hinkle, J., & Cheever, K. (2010), pp. 839–840.

139. ANSWER: 0.5
The dosage strength on the label is 1.25 mg/mL. The desired dose is 0.625 mg. Use a proportion formula to calculate the correct amount to administer. Multiply the outside values and then the inside values and solve for X.

1.25 mg : 1 mL :: 0.625 mg : X mL

1.25 X = 0.625

X = 0.5

TEST-TAKING TIP: Recognize that the dose to be administered is less than the dose supplied. Double-check the calculations if the amount is greater than 0.5 mL.

Content Area: Adult Health; **Category of Health Alteration:** Cardiac Management; **Integrated Processes:** Nursing Process Implementation; **Client Need:** Physiological Integrity/Pharmacological and Parenteral Therapies/Dosage Calculation; **Cognitive Level:** Application; **Reference:** Pickar, G., & Abernethy, A. (2008), p. 46.

Test 16: Adult Health: Endocrine Management

140. A client with diabetes mellitus shows the device illustrated to a nurse. Which statement made by the client should indicate to the nurse that additional teaching is needed?

1. "I take my insulin pump off when I shower and sometimes when I exercise."
2. "I count the number of carbohydrates (CHOs) eaten and then set the pump to deliver the required amount of insulin."
3. "Today I attached the pump to my waistband, but I usually wear it in the pocket of my pants."
4. "Because I don't want an infection, I have been changing the needle and tubing once a week."

141. A nurse is preparing to administer the bedtime dose of insulin aspart (Novolog) to a 19-year-old client who has type 1 diabetes mellitus. The client's blood glucose level is 225 mg/dL. According to the sliding scale presented, how many units of insulin should the nurse administer?

_____ units (Record your answer as a whole number.)

Glucose Level mg/dL	Mealtime Units of Aspart Insulin for Glucose Level	HS Dose of Aspart Insulin for Glucose Level
60–69	−3 and call	−3
70–79	−2	−2
80–89	−1	−1
90–130	0	0
131–150	2	0
151–200	4	2
201–250	6	3
251–300	7	4
Greater than 300 call		

140. ANSWER: 4.
The needle and catheter tubing should be changed every 3 days because the tubing or needle can become occluded resulting in unexpected disruptions in the flow of insulin. The pump is easily disconnected and can be removed for limited periods to shower or during exercise. When a pump is used, insulin is delivered by a subcutaneous infusion at a basal rate. To metabolize the CHOs from a consumed meal, the client calculates an additional dose of insulin to deliver by a bolus infusion from the pump. The pump can be worn either on a belt or in a pocket. Some women wear the pump tucked into the front or side of the bra or attached to a garter belt on the thigh.

TEST-TAKING TIP: Read each option carefully. Select an option that can increase the risk of the insulin infusion system malfunctioning.

Content Area: Adult Health; **Category of Health Alteration:** Endocrine Management; **Integrated Processes:** Caring; Teaching and Learning; **Client Need:** Physiological Integrity/Pharmacological and Parenteral Therapies/Medication Administration; **Cognitive Level:** Analysis; **Reference:** Smeltzer, S., Bare, B., Hinkle, J., & Cheever, K. (2010), pp. 1212–1213; **EBP Reference:** Barnard, K., Lloyd, C., & Skinner, T. (2007). Systematic literature review: Quality of life associated with insulin pump use in type 1 diabetes. *Diabetic Medicine*, 24(6), 607–617.

141. ANSWER: 3
Three units of aspart insulin are administered if the glucose level ranges between 201 and 250 mg/dL. The bedtime/overnight target range for adolescents 13 to 19 years is 90 to 150 mg/dL, whereas the before-meal target range is 90 to 130 mg/dL—thus the differences between mealtime and bedtime HS dosing.

TEST-TAKING TIP: Carefully read what the question is asking. Be sure to note the HS dose of the insulin. Insulin order sheets frequently contain all insulin orders, and the nurse must determine the correct amount based on the client's glucose level and the orders.

Content Area: Adult Health; **Category of Health Alteration:** Endocrine Management; **Integrated Processes:** Nursing Process Planning; **Client Need:** Physiological Integrity/Pharmacological and Parenteral Therapies/Dosage Calculation; **Cognitive Level:** Analysis; **References:** Ball, J., & Bindler, R. (2008), pp. 1228–1229; Lewis, S., Heitkemper, M., Dirksen, S., Bucher, L., Camera, I. (2011), pp. 1227–1228.

142. A client is receiving treatment for syndrome of inappropriate antidiuretic hormone (SIADH). The nurse evaluates that treatment has been effective when which findings are noted? **Select all that apply.**

1. Decrease in weight
2. Increase in serum osmolality
3. Decrease in urine osmolality
4. Increase in blood pressure (BP)
5. Increase in serum sodium
6. Absence of muscle twitching and muscle cramps

143. A nurse is assessing a client newly diagnosed with hypothyroidism. Which findings should the nurse expect? **Select all that apply.**

1. Complaints of feeling cold
2. An enlarged thyroid gland
3. Fine hand tremors
4. Thick, brittle nails
5. Weight gain
6. Irritability

142. ANSWER: 1, 2, 3, 5, 6.
Decreased weight, increased serum osmolality, decreased urine osmolality, increased serum sodium, and an absence of muscle twitching and muscle cramps indicate that treatment is effective. In SIADH, the posterior pituitary gland increases the secretion of antidiuretic hormone (vasopressin), which increases water reabsorption in the renal tubules and consequently increases intravascular fluid volume resulting in dilutional hyponatremia and decreased serum osmolality. The water reabsorption causes the urine to be concentrated (increased urine osmolality). Fluid retention causes weight gain and increased blood pressure. Hyponatremia causes muscle cramps, weakness, and twitching. Effective treatment should result in a reduction of the manifestations of SIADH, thus the BP should decrease, not increase.

TEST-TAKING TIP: The key words are "effective treatment." Think about the signs and symptoms of SIADH. Effective treatment should result in a reduction of these.

Content Area: Adult Health; **Category of Health Alteration:** Endocrine Management; **Integrated Processes:** Nursing Process Evaluation; **Client Need:** Physiological Integrity/Physiological Adaptation/Alterations in Body Systems; **Cognitive Level:** Analysis; **Reference:** Lewis, S., Heitkemper, M., Dirksen, S., Bucher, L., & Camera, I. (2011), pp. 1256–1258, 1795–1798.

143. ANSWER: 1, 4, 5.
There is an insufficient amount of circulating thyroid hormone in hypothyroidism. This insufficiency produces slowing of metabolic activity with cardiovascular, respiratory, gastrointestinal, integumentary, musculoskeletal, nervous, and reproductive system effects. Feeling cold and weight gain are among the effects. Thick, brittle nails occur from metabolite build-up as a result of the decreased cellular energy. An enlarged thyroid gland, fine hand tremors, and irritability are associated with hyperthyroidism (too much circulating thyroid hormone).

TEST-TAKING TIP: Focus on the options that suggest reduced metabolic activity.

Content Area: Adult Health; **Category of Health Alteration:** Endocrine Management; **Integrated Processes:** Nursing Process Assessment; **Client Need:** Physiological Integrity/Reduction of Risk Potential/System Specific Assessments; **Cognitive Level:** Application; **References:** Lewis, S., Heitkemper, M., Dirksen, S., Bucher, L., & Camera, I. (2011), p. 1264; Smeltzer, S., Bare, B., Hinkle, J., & Cheever, K. (2010), pp. 1272–1275.

144. A nurse is developing a care plan for a client diagnosed with Cushing's syndrome. Which nursing diagnoses should the nurse document in the client's plan of care? **Select all that apply.**

1. Hyperthermia related to suppression of adrenal cortical hormone
2. Disturbed thought processes related to mood swings, irritability, and depression
3. Risk for infection related to altered protein metabolism and inflammatory response
4. Self-care deficit related to weakness, fatigue, muscle wasting, and altered sleep patterns
5. Disturbed body image related to altered physical appearance and impaired sexual functioning
6. Risk for myxedema coma related to medication nonadherence secondary to depression

145. A nurse completed an assessment for a client diagnosed with Addison's disease. Which findings indicate that the client is being treated effectively? **Select all that apply.**

1. Blood pressure 120/80 mm Hg
2. Client states the purpose of hydrocortisone (Solu-Cortef)
3. Denies muscle weakness and fatigue
4. Serum glucose 90 mg/dL
5. Serum sodium 128 mEq/L
6. Serum potassium 5.9 mEq/L

144. ANSWER: 2, 3, 4, 5.

The overproduction of adrenal cortical hormone that occurs in Cushing's syndrome produces ophthalmic, cardiovascular, endocrine, metabolic, immune, skeletal, GI, muscular, dermatological, and psychiatric changes. Cushing's syndrome occurs from an overproduction (not suppression) of adrenal cortical hormone. Myxedema coma is associated with hypothyroidism.

TEST-TAKING TIP: Carefully read each option to determine if the nursing diagnosis and related parts of the nursing diagnosis are associated with Cushing's syndrome. Eliminate options 1 and 6.

Content Area: Adult Health; **Category of Health Alteration:** Endocrine Management; **Integrated Processes:** Communication and Documentation; **Client Need:** Safe and Effective Care Environment/Management of Care/Continuity of Care; **Cognitive Level:** Analysis; **Reference:** Smeltzer, S., Bare, B., Hinkle, J., & Cheever, K. (2010), p. 1281.

145. ANSWER: 1, 3, 4.

Addison's disease (adrenocortical insufficiency) is characterized by hypotension, muscle weakness, hypoglycemia, hyponatremia, hyperkalemia, as well as other signs and symptoms. A reversal of these symptoms indicates treatment is effective. Normal serum sodium is 135–145 mEq/L; hyponatremia is still present. The normal serum potassium is 3.5–5.0 mEq/L; hyperkalemia is present.

TEST-TAKING TIP: The key words are "treated effectively." Select the options in which the finding is normal but would be abnormal in Addison's disease.

Content Area: Adult Health; **Category of Health Alteration:** Endocrine Management; **Integrated Processes:** Nursing Process Evaluation; **Client Need:** Physiological Integrity/Physiological Adaptation/Alterations in Body Systems; **Cognitive Level:** Analysis; **Reference:** Smeltzer, S., Bare, B., Hinkle, J., & Cheever, K. (2010), p. 1279.

Test 17: Adult Health: Gastrointestinal Management

146. A nurse is making a home visit to a client who had an esophagogastrostomy 3 weeks previously for esophageal cancer. After reviewing the client's laboratory report, which nursing diagnosis should be the nurse's priority?

Serum Laboratory Report	Client Value	Normal Values
BUN	2	5–25 mg
Creatinine	1.2	0.5–1.5 mg/dL
Na	140	135–145 mEqL
K	4.5	3.5–5.3 mEq/L
Cl	99	95–105 mEq/L
CO_2	23	22–30 mEq/L
Hgb	10	13.5–17 g/dL
Hct	30%	40%–54%
Albumin	2.6	3.5–5.0 g/dL
WBC	5,000	4,500–10,000/µL or mm^3

1. Altered nutrition less than body requirements
2. Ineffective airway clearance
3. Acute pain
4. Risk for injury

147. A client, who had a laparoscopic cholecystectomy the previous day, is now calling a clinic to report the development of right shoulder pain. Which advice should the nurse give to the client? **Select all that apply.**

1. Come immediately to the clinic.
2. Sit upright in bed or in a chair.
3. Apply a heating pad to the shoulder for 15 minutes every hour.
4. Do range of motion (ROM) exercises on the right shoulder three times a day.
5. Eliminate the fat in your diet today and then gradually add fat back into your diet.

146. ANSWER: 1.
Decreased serum albumin levels are a sign of malnutrition, and low hemoglobin levels can be a result of anemia from decreased iron intake. Maintaining adequate nutrition after esophageal surgery can be difficult because of the location of the surgery. There is no indication that pain control and risk for injury are problems. Ineffective airway clearance might be evidenced by elevated white blood cells (WBCs). However, this client's WBCs are within the normal range.

TEST-TAKING TIP: Note the type of surgery that the client experienced and the likely long-term complications of that surgery. If uncertain, associate the GI tract with nutrition.

Content Area: Adult Health; **Category of Health Alteration:** Gastrointestinal Management; **Integrated Processes:** Nursing Process Analysis; **Client Need:** Physiological Integrity/Reduction of Risk Potential/Laboratory Values; **Cognitive Level:** Analysis; **References:** Ignatavicius, D., & Workman, M. (2010), pp. 1259–1260; Kee, J. (2009), pp. 84–86, 96–100, 106–108, 146–148, 220–224, 335–340, 385–388, 437–439.

147. ANSWER: 2, 3.
The nurse's advice should be to sit upright and apply heat to help control this pain. During a laparoscopic cholecystectomy, the abdomen is insufflated with carbon dioxide to assist in inserting the laparoscope and to aid in visualization. The carbon dioxide will migrate to the diaphragm and cause nerve irritation and shoulder pain. There is no need for an emergent clinic visit. ROM exercises are not supported by the literature to decrease this type of pain. Although fat should be gradually added back into the diet if the client had fat intolerance before surgery, the right shoulder pain is from the gas used for inflation and is unrelated to the diet.

TEST-TAKING TIP: Remember that the gas used to inflate the abdominal area produces the pain. Use this information to eliminate options.

Content Area: Adult Health; **Category of Health Alteration:** Gastrointestinal Management; **Integrated Processes:** Nursing Process Implementation; **Client Need:** Physiological Integrity/Basic Care and Comfort/Nonpharmacological Comfort Interventions; **Cognitive Level:** Application; **Reference:** Smeltzer, S., Bare, B., Hinkle, J., & Cheever, K. (2008), p. 1181.

148. A client with a known peptic ulcer is admitted to an emergency department after vomiting a large amount of coffee ground emesis. Vital signs are BP: 100/60 mm Hg; P: 100 beats per minute; RR: 24 breaths per minute; and temperature: 99.0°F (37.2°C). Which interventions should a nurse anticipate in the client's initial collaborative plan of care? **Select all that apply.**

1. Administering intravenous (IV) fluids
2. Inserting a nasogastric (NG) tube and placing it on suction
3. Having the client sign a consent for emergency surgery
4. Positioning the client in Trendelenburg's position
5. Administering a proton pump inhibitor
6. Limiting the client's diet to bland foods only

149. Four hours following an abdominal Nissen fundoplication for repair of a hiatal hernia, a client has yellow-green drainage in the nasogastric (NG) tube and absent bowel sounds. Which actions by the nurse are most appropriate? **Select all that apply.**

1. Notify the surgeon immediately.
2. Document the findings.
3. Reposition the NG tube.
4. Offer a clear liquid diet.
5. Continue to monitor the client.

148. ANSWER: 1, 2, 5.
The client experiencing GI bleeding is at risk for hemorrhagic shock, which should be treated with IV fluids. IV access is needed for IV medications. NG suction clears the stomach of blood and acid, protects the client from aspiration, allows monitoring of amount and type of bleeding, and prevents nausea and vomiting. Proton pump inhibitors raise the gastric pH to a level that can support clotting. Options 3, 4, and 6 are incorrect because immediate surgery is not recommended. Most episodes of GI bleeding stop spontaneously; if not, bleeding control is attempted first per endoscopy and not surgery. There is a serious risk of aspiration with hematemesis, so the client should be placed with the head of bed elevated to 45 degrees. All food is contraindicated in the presence of nausea and vomiting.

TEST-TAKING TIP: Coffee ground emesis indicates slow gastric bleeding, which initially can be treated conservatively.

Content Area: Adult Health; **Category of Health Alteration:** Gastrointestinal Management; **Integrated Processes:** Nursing Process Implementation; **Client Need:** Physiological Integrity/Physiological Adaptation/Medical Emergencies;
Cognitive Level: Application; **Reference:** Smeltzer, S., Bare, B., Hinkle, J., & Cheever, K. (2010), pp. 1047–1054; **EBP Reference:** Wang, Y., Pan, T., Wang, Q., & Guo, Z. (2009). Additional bedtime H_2-receptor antagonist for the control of nocturnal gastric acid breakthrough. *Cochrane Database of Systematic Reviews*, Issue 4, Art. No.: CD004275. DOI: 10.1002/14651858.CD004275.pub3.

149. ANSWER: 2, 5.
None of the findings are unexpected 4 hours after esophageal surgery, so the only actions necessary are documentation and continued monitoring. There is no reason to notify the surgeon, and the NG tube should not be repositioned because of the potential to disrupt suture lines. Oral fluids are not given until peristalsis returns.

TEST-TAKING TIP: Consider that the findings are expected after upper gastrointestinal surgery.

Content Area: Adult Health; **Category of Health Alteration:** Gastrointestinal Management; **Integrated Processes:** Nursing Process Implementation; **Client Need:** Physiological Integrity/Physiologic Adaptation/Illness Management;
Cognitive Level: Analysis; **References:** Ignatavicius, D., & Workman, M. (2010), p. 1254; Lewis, S., Heitkemper, M., Dirksen, S., Bucher, L., & Camera, I. (2011), pp. 997–998.

150. A nurse is assessing a client newly diagnosed with Crohn's disease. Which findings should the nurse associate with Crohn's disease? **Select all that apply.**

1. Weight gain
2. Crampy abdominal pains
3. Chronic constipation
4. Steatorrhea
5. Anemia

151. A nurse is to initiate tube feedings for a client who has gastrostomy tube. Into which tube on the illustration should the nurse plan to administer the feedings?

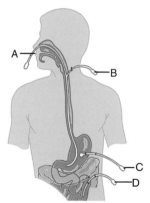

1. A
2. B
3. C
4. D

150. ANSWER: 2, 4, 5.
Crohn's disease is a subacute and chronic inflammation of the gastrointestinal (GI) tract that extends through all layers. Lesions, fistulas, fissure, abscesses, scar tissue, and granulomas develop. The scar tissue and granulomas interfere with the ability of the intestine to transport products of upper intestinal digestion through the constricted lumen resulting in crampy abdominal pains. Disrupted absorption causes steatorrhea (excessive fat in the stools), chronic nutritional deficits, and anemia. Weight loss (not gain) and diarrhea (not constipation) are other symptoms of Crohn's disease.

TEST-TAKING TIP: Eliminate options that do not pertain to malabsorption.

Content Area: Adult Health; Category of Health Alteration: Gastrointestinal Management; Integrated Processes: Nursing Process Assessment; Client Need: Physiological Integrity/Physiological Adaptation/Alterations in Body Systems; Cognitive Level: Application; Reference: Smeltzer, S., Bare, B., Hinkle, J., & Cheever, K. (2010), pp. 1082–1083.

151. ANSWER: 3.
A gastrostomy tube (Line C) is placed surgically through an abdominal incision into the stomach. The distal end of the tube is secured to the anterior gastric wall, a tunnel is created, and then the proximal end of the tube is brought through the abdomen to form a permanent stoma. Line A is a nasogastric tube, which ends in the stomach. Line B is an esophagostomy tube. Line D is a jejunostomy tube, which is placed similarly to the gastrostomy tube, but the distal end extends beyond the pylorus into the jejunum.

TEST-TAKING TIP: Apply knowledge of medical terminology to select the correct option. "Gastro" pertains to the stomach.

Content Area: Adult Health; Category of Health Alteration: Gastrointestinal Management; Integrated Processes: Nursing Process Planning; Client Need: Physiological Integrity/Basic Care and Comfort/Nutrition and Oral Hydration; Cognitive Level: Application; Reference: Smeltzer, S., Bare, B., Hinkle, J., & Cheever, K. (2010), pp. 1031–1032.

152. A nurse is teaching a client who underwent a Bilroth I gastroduo-denostomy. Place an X on the illustration that the nurse should use when teaching this client.

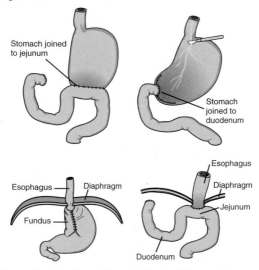

153. A nurse has developed the goal of maintaining weight appropriate for height for a client with anorexia as a result of acute hepatitis. Which interventions should the nurse add to the client's plan of care? **Select all that apply.**

1. Serve larger quantities of food in the morning than at the supper meal.
2. Include carbonated beverages in the client's diet.
3. Provide mouth care before meals.
4. Serve hot and spicy foods.
5. Avoid the use of antiemetics.
6. Offer several smaller meals rather than three large meals.

152. ANSWER:

In a Bilroth I procedure, the distal portion of the stomach is removed and the remaining portion is sutured to the duodenum. In Bilroth II, the remaining portion of the stomach is sutured to the proximal jejunum. The third illustration is of a Nissen fundoplication for a hiatal hernia repair. The last illustration is a total gastrectomy in which the stomach is removed and the esophagus is sutured to the jejunum.

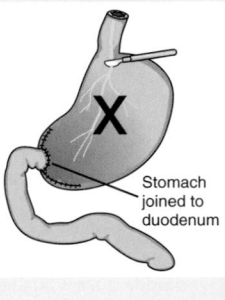

Stomach joined to duodenum

TEST-TAKING TIP: Select an option that shows removal of a portion of the stomach. Use a memory cue to differentiate Bilroth I from Bilroth II. The "d" in duodenum is before the "j" in jejunum in the alphabet; anatomically, the duodenum is before the jejunum.

Content Area: Adult Health; **Category of Health Alteration:** Gastrointestinal Management; **Integrated Processes:** Teaching and Learning; **Client Need:** Physiological Integrity/Physiological Adaptation/Pathophysiology; **Cognitive Level:** Application; **Reference:** Smeltzer, S., Bare, B., Hinkle, J., & Cheever, K. (2010), pp. 1012–1013, 1051–1052, 1058.

153. ANSWER: 1, 2, 3, 6.

Clients with hepatitis often find that their anorexia is more pronounced in the evening than in the morning and thus they are able to eat a larger breakfast rather than a larger supper. Carbonated beverages and frequent mouth care promote increase in appetite. Several smaller meals are better tolerated than less frequent larger meals. Very hot or very cold foods are not well tolerated because these increase nausea. Antiemetics should be used (rather than avoided) to decrease nausea before meals.

TEST-TAKING TIP: Focus on basic nursing interventions that promote appetite in a client. This should allow elimination of options 4 and 5.

Content Area: Adult Health; **Category of Health Alteration:** Infectious Disease; **Integrated Processes:** Nursing Process Planning; **Client Need:** Physiological Integrity/Basic Care and Comfort/Nutrition and Oral Hydration; **Cognitive Level:** Application; **Reference:** Osborn, S., Wraa, C., & Watson, A. (2010), pp. 1431–1434.

Test 18: Adult Health: Hematological and Oncological Management

154. A nurse admits a 24-year-old female client with suspected Hodgkin's lymphoma. When preparing the client for a physician's examination and diagnostic tests, which statements to the client are correct? **Select all that apply.**

1. "The routine CBC always includes an analysis for B lymphocytes. So you are finished with lab work."
2. "The enlarged painless lymph nodes in your neck usually are the first to appear, so the physician will be palpating lymph nodes throughout your body."
3. "The physician will be palpating your left upper quadrant for an enlarged spleen."
4. "A lymph node biopsy will be performed; the diagnosis can be confirmed if there are Reed-Sternberg cells."
5. "You will have a chest x-ray and CT scan of the chest and abdomen to determine if there is lymph tissue enlargement in these areas."
6. "A pregnancy test will be performed to check for pregnancy. Some treatments would not be initiated if you are pregnant."

155. Which findings should a nurse expect when assessing a client diagnosed with acute myeloid leukemia (AML)? **Select all that apply.**

1. Temperature 102.2°F (39°C)
2. Hyperplasia of the gums
3. Bone pain rated at 7 out of 10 on a numeric scale
4. Rebound tenderness right lower abdomen
5. Weakness and fatigue

154. ANSWER: 2, 3, 4, 5, 6.
The correct statements include informing the client about the physical examination of palpating the lymph nodes and the spleen to determine tissue involvement. The diagnostic tests include a lymph node biopsy, and the presence of Reed-Sternberg cells can confirm the diagnosis. Chest x-ray and a CT scan can help determine the extent of involvement. If the client is pregnant, chemotherapy and radiation would not be initiated because the developing fetus would be subjected to their effects. Option 1 is incorrect. A specialized test, in addition to the complete blood count (CBC), is done to analyze for B lymphocytes.

TEST-TAKING TIP: Examine each option carefully. Think about the laboratory results obtained in a CBC. Consider that a CBC is routinely performed whereas persons are not routinely tested for Hodgkin's lymphoma.

Content Area: Adult Health; **Category of Health Alteration:** Hematological and Oncological Management; **Integrated Processes:** Teaching and Learning; **Client Need:** Safe and Effective Care Environment/Management of Care/Continuity of Care/Physiological Integrity/Reduction of Risk Potential/Diagnostic Tests; **Cognitive Level:** Application; **Reference:** Smeltzer, S., Bare, B., Hinkle, J., & Cheever, K. (2010), pp. 941–943.

155. ANSWER: 1, 2, 3, 5.
Signs and symptoms of AML result from insufficient production of normal blood cells. Fever and infection result from neutropenia. The proliferation of leukemic cells produces gum hyperplasia, and expansion of bone marrow produces bone pain. Weakness and fatigue result from anemia. Rebound tenderness in the right lower abdomen could be indicative of appendicitis.

TEST-TAKING TIP: Select options that relate to insufficient production of normal blood cells.

Content Area: Adult Health; **Category of Health Alteration:** Hematological and Oncological Management; **Integrated Processes:** Nursing Process Assessment; **Client Need:** Physiological Integrity/Physiological Adaptation/Alterations in Body Systems; **Cognitive Level:** Application; **Reference:** Smeltzer, S., Bare, B., Hinkle, J., & Cheever, K. (2008), p. 933.

156. A nurse is caring for four clients. In which order should the nurse assess the clients based on each client's potential for bleeding? Place each client in the correct numerical order (1–4) based on the risk for bleeding.

_____ 1. Client with a platelet count of 50,000/mm³
_____ 2. Client with a platelet count of 18,000/mm³
_____ 3. Client receiving warfarin (Coumadin) and the prothrombin time (PT) is 12 seconds
_____ 4. Client receiving a heparin infusion and the activated partial thromboplastin time (aPTT) is 52 seconds

157. A clinic nurse is caring for a male client who has been receiving radiation to the mantle field for Hodgkin's lymphoma. Which common side effects of radiation therapy should a nurse monitor for this client? **Select all that apply.**

1. Urticaria and neuropathy
2. Cardiotoxicity and elevated blood pressure
3. Dry mouth (xerostomia) and dysphagia
4. Angioedema and nephrotoxicity
5. Stomatitis and loss of chest hair

156. ANSWER: 2, 1, 4, 3.
The client with a platelet count of 18,000/mm³ has a severe risk for spontaneous bleeding. Platelets are essential to blood clotting. Normal platelet counts are 150,000 to 400,000/mm³. The client with a platelet count of 50,000/mm³ has a moderate risk for bleeding. Next, the nurse should assess the client on a heparin infusion. The aPTT is used to evaluate the effectiveness of heparin. A therapeutic range is 1.5–2.5 times baseline values (20–39 seconds). An adjustment of the heparin dose is required for aPTT less than 50 seconds. Last assessed is the client receiving warfarin. The normal PT is 9.5–12 seconds. PT is used to monitor the effectiveness of warfarin as an anticoagulant. This value is nontherapeutic.

TEST-TAKING TIP: Identify the normal laboratory values and rank these options last.

Content Area: Adult Health; **Category of Health Alteration:** Hematological and Oncological Management; **Integrated Processes:** Nursing Process Planning; **Client Need:** Safe and Effective Care Environment/Management of Care/Establishing Priorities; **Cognitive Level:** Analysis; **Reference:** Smeltzer, S., Bare, B., Hinkle, J., & Cheever, K. (2010), pp. 375, 706.

157. ANSWER: 3, 5.
Radiation to the mantle field is radiation to the chest wall, mediastinum, axilla, and neck region. Dry mouth, dysphagia, stomatitis, and loss of chest hair occur frequently with mantle field irradiation. Urticaria, neuropathy, cardiotoxicity, elevated blood pressure, angioedema, and nephrotoxicity are side effects of chemotherapeutic agents.

TEST-TAKING TIP: Think about the effects and location of irradiation and use the process of elimination. Options 1 and 4 (kidneys and peripheral neuropathy) are outside the areas of the radiation treatment. Since cardiac side effects are rare, options 3 and 5 remain the only viable options.

Content Area: Adult Health; **Category of Health Alteration:** Hematological and Oncological Management; **Integrated Processes:** Nursing Process Assessment; **Client Need:** Physiological Integrity/Physiological Adaptation/Alterations in Body Systems; **Cognitive Level:** Analysis; **Reference:** Smeltzer, S., Bare, B., Hinkle, J., & Cheever, K. (2010), pp. 350–351.

158. A client is experiencing stomatitis. Which interventions should a nurse include in the client's plan of care? **Select all that apply.**

1. Remove dentures except for meals.
2. Have client gargle a preferred alcohol-based mouthwash brought from home.
3. Apply water-soluble lip lubricant.
4. Use toothettes soaked with saline solution and viscous lidocaine for oral care.
5. Avoid foods that are spicy and hard to chew.

159. A nurse is preparing to care for a client who had a pneumonectomy for treatment of lung cancer. Which illustration reflects the nurse's critical thinking about the extent of the surgery performed? Place an X on the appropriate illustration.

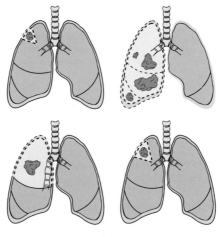

158. ANSWER: 1, 3, 4, 5.
Removing dentures prevents trauma from ill-fitting dentures. Lip lubricant promotes comfort. Oral care with saline and viscous lidocaine alleviates pain, increases a sense of well-being, and promotes participation in oral hygiene and nutritional intake. Avoiding spicy foods prevents local trauma. Alcohol-based mouthwashes are drying to oral tissues and potentiate breakdown.

TEST-TAKING TIP: Eliminate any options that will dry oral tissues.

Content Area: Adult Health; **Category of Health Alteration:** Hematological and Oncological Management; **Integrated Processes:** Nursing Process Implementation; **Client Need:** Physiological Integrity/Reduction of Risk Potential/Therapeutic Procedures; **Cognitive Level:** Application; **Reference:** Smeltzer, S., Bare, B., Hinkle, J., & Cheever, K. (2010), pp. 367–368; **EBP Reference:** Clarkson, J., Worthington, H., & Eden, O. (2008). Interventions for preventing oral candidiasis for patients with cancer receiving treatment. *Cochrane Database of Systematic Reviews*, 3. Retrieved from www.cochrane.org/reviews/en/ab003807.html.

159. ANSWER:
A pneumonectomy is removal of an entire lung and is performed chiefly for cancer when the lesion cannot be removed by a less extensive procedure. The first illustration is a segmental resection. Bronchopulmonary segments are subdivisions of the lung that function as individual units. The third illustration is a lobectomy in which only a lobe of the lung is removed. The last illustration is a wedge resection where a small well-circumscribed lesion is removed without regard for the location of the inter-segmental planes.

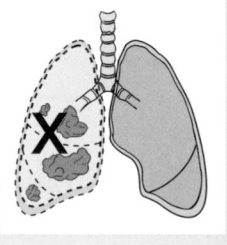

TEST-TAKING TIP: Select the option that is most extensive.

Content Area: Adult Health; **Category of Health Alteration:** Hematological and Oncological Management; **Integrated Processes:** Nursing Process Analysis; **Client Need:** Physiological Integrity/Physiological Adaptation/Alterations in Body Systems; **Cognitive Level:** Application; **Reference:** Smeltzer, S., Bare, B., Hinkle, J., & Cheever, K. (2010), p. 665.

160. A nurse, analyzing a serum laboratory report for a client receiving chemotherapy for cancer, determines that the client has pancytopenia. Which findings in the laboratory report prompted the nurse to reach this conclusion? **Select all that apply.**

1. Decreased platelets
2. Decreased white blood cell count (WBC)
3. Decreased red blood cell count (RBC)
4. Decreased partial thromboplastin time (PTT)
5. Decreased prothrombin time (PT)

161. A nurse cares for a client experiencing severe nausea from an acoustic neuroma. A dose of promethazine (Phenergan) 25 mg IM is ordered. The 10 mL medication vial contains 50 mg per 1 mL. How many milliliters (mL) of the medication should the nurse prepare for injection?

____ mL (Record your answer to the nearest tenth.)

160. ANSWER: 1, 2, 3.
Pancytopenia is a simultaneous reduction in all cellular elements in the blood including platelets (thrombocytopenia), WBCs (leukopenia), and anemia (RBCs). The PTT and PT are measures of coagulation and not cellular elements.

TEST-TAKING TIP: Apply knowledge of medical terminology: "pan-" means all, "cyto-" pertains to cell, and "-penia" means decreased. Eliminate options 4 and 5 because these do not pertain to the cells but are a measurement of coagulation.

Content Area: Adult Health; **Category of Health Alteration:** Hematological and Oncological Management; **Integrated Processes:** Nursing Process Evaluation; **Client Need:** Physiological Integrity/Reduction of Risk Potential/Laboratory Values; **Cognitive Level:** Analysis; **References:** Smeltzer, S., Bare, B., Hinkle, J., & Cheever, K. (2010), pp. 903, 917.

161. ANSWER: 0.5
Use a proportion formula to calculate the dose:

50 mg : 1 mL :: 25 mg: X mL

Multiply the extremes (outside values) and means (inside values) and solve for X.

$50\,X = 25$

$X = 25/50$

$X = 0.5$ mL

TEST-TAKING TIP: Focus on the information in the question. You should be able to think this problem through and recognize that 25 is $\frac{1}{2}$ of 50.

Content Area: Adult Health; **Category of Health Alteration:** Hematologic and Oncologic Management; **Integrated Processes:** Nursing Process Implementation; **Client Need:** Physiological Integrity/Pharmacological and Parenteral Therapies/Dosage Calculation; **Cognitive Level:** Application; **Reference:** Pickar, G., & Abernethy, A. (2008), p. 46.

Test 19: Adult Health: Integumentary Management and Other Health Alterations

162. A nurse is explaining to a coworker the layer of tissue burned during a second-degree burn. Which location should the nurse identify to the coworker?

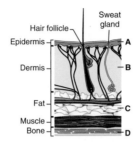

1. A
2. B
3. C
4. D

163. A nurse is estimating the extent of a client's burn injury. Using the "rule of nines," what percentage of the client's body surface should the nurse determine has been burned?

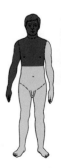

_____ percent (Record your answer as a whole number.)

162. ANSWER: 2.
A second-degree burn involves all of the epidermis and some of the dermis (also called partial-thickness burn) and may be characterized by blisters or penetrate as far down as the dermis. A first-degree burn involves only the epidermis (A) with only erythema and minor microscopic changes. A third-degree burn (C or D) involves subcutaneous tissue (also called full-thickness burn) and may go down to bone or fascia.

TEST-TAKING TIP: Note the keywords "second-degree burn" and remember a second-degree burn involves the first and second layer of the skin.

Content Area: Adult Health; **Category of Health Alteration:** Integumentary Management and Other Health Alterations; **Integrated Processes:** Teaching and Learning; **Client Need:** Physiological Integrity/Physiological Adaptation/ Pathophysiology; **Cognitive Level:** Analysis; **Reference:** Black, J., & Hokanson Hawks, J. (2009), pp. 1243–1245.

163. ANSWER: 36
Using the "rule of nines," the head and neck is 9%, the right arm is 9%, and the chest is 18%. The total body surface area burned is 36%.

TEST-TAKING TIP: If unsure, recall that the largest body surface area is 18%.

Content Area: Adult Health; **Category of Health Alteration:** Integumentary Management and other Health Alterations; **Integrated Processes:** Nursing Process Analysis; **Client Need:** Physiological Integrity/Physiological Adaptation/Alterations in Body Systems; **Cognitive Level:** Analysis; **Reference:** Smeltzer, S., Bare, B., Hinkle, J., & Cheever, K. (2010), p. 1781.

164. Which statements to a nurse indicate that the client has achieved expected outcomes after a burn injury? **Select all that apply.**

1. "I used to wake up almost every hour with nightmares of being burned, but now it only occurs once or twice a night."
2. "How do you like my new wig? My husband helped me select it. I always wanted blond hair, and I think it makes me look terrific!"
3. "Now that I am in outpatient rehabilitation, I have been socializing a lot more with my friends. I even joined a Yoga class."
4. "I wish I had not picked up that burning pan from the stove to throw it outdoors; but it was such an instant reaction."
5. "I haven't been able to think about returning to work yet; I am so busy with my daily physical therapy and learning how to do the dressing changes for myself."

165. Which manifestations should a nurse associate with the development of staphylococcal cellulitis?

1. Inflammation
2. Lymphadenopathy
3. Cool to touch
4. Localized edema
5. Pallor
6. Pain

164. ANSWER: 2, 3.
The statement in option 2 shows that the client has adapted to an altered body image and has an improved self-concept. The statement in option 3 also supports that the client has adapted to an altered body image and shows a gradual increase in tolerance and endurance in physical activities. The statement in option 1 indicates that the client is progressing toward the outcome of reporting absence of nightmares but has not yet fully achieved the outcome. The statement in option 4 suggests the client's ability to talk about the event, but does not show achievement of an expected outcome. The statement in option 5 also shows some achievement in the outcome in the ability to perform wound care but has not yet achieved the outcome.

TEST-TAKING TIP: Eliminate statements in which the outcomes are only partially met (options 1, 4, and 5).

Content Area: Adult Health; **Category of Health Alteration:** Integument and Other Health Alterations; **Integrated Processes:** Nursing Process Evaluation; **Client Need:** Safe and Effective Care Environment/Management of Care/Continuity of Care; **Cognitive Level:** Analysis; **Reference:** Smeltzer, S., Bare, B., Hinkle, J., & Cheever, K. (2010), pp. 1748–1751.

165. ANSWER: 1, 2, 4, 6.
Cellulitis is inflammation of the skin and subcutaneous tissue from an infection with clinical signs and symptoms of lymphadenopathy, localized edema, and pain. Cool to touch and pallor are not signs of inflammation, but could indicate impaired circulation from swelling.

TEST-TAKING TIP: Focus on the key words of "most likely" and "cellulitis." Think about changes that occur with inflammation. Eliminate options 3 and 5 because these relate to impaired circulation.

Content Area: Adult Health; **Category of Health Alteration:** Integument and Other Health Alterations; **Integrated Processes:** Nursing Process Assessment; **Client Need:** Physiological Integrity/Physiological Adaptation/Alterations in Body Systems; **Cognitive Level:** Application; **Reference:** Black, J., & Hawks, J. (2009), pp. 1225–1226.

Test 20: Adult Health: Musculoskeletal Management

166. A nurse is evaluating a client's ability to perform quadriceps muscle-setting exercises. Place each step in the numerical order (1–6) that the client should demonstrate performing these exercises correctly.

_____ 1. Holds the position for 5 to 10 seconds
_____ 2. Positions supine in bed with legs extended
_____ 3. Relaxes the quadriceps muscles
_____ 4. Contracts the anterior thigh muscles
_____ 5. Repeats the exercise nine more times
_____ 6. Pushes the knee back onto the mattress

167. Which instructions should a nurse provide when teaching a client conservative management and measures to slow the progression of osteoarthritis of the right knee? **Select all that apply.**

1. Reduce weight by consuming a reduced calorie diet.
2. Begin a progressive walking program.
3. Apply cold to the knee joint for swelling, or heat for comfort.
4. Obtain a prescription for narcotic analgesics for pain control.
5. Stand as much as possible for completing work and other household activities.

166. ANSWER: 2, 4, 6, 1, 3, 5.
First, the client should be positioned supine in bed with the legs extended. Next, the client should contract the anterior thigh muscles and then push the knee back onto the mattress. This position should be held for 5 to 10 seconds, and then the client relaxes the quadriceps muscles. Finally, the client should repeat the exercise nine more times.

TEST-TAKING TIP: Attempt to perform muscle exercises and then look for the options to mimic your sequence of actions.

Content Area: Adult Health; **Category of Health Alteration:** Musculoskeletal Management; **Integrated Processes:** Nursing Process Evaluation; **Client Need:** Physiological Integrity/Basic Care and Comfort/Mobility/Immobility; **Cognitive Level:** Application; **Reference:** Smeltzer, S., Bare, B., Hinkle, J., & Cheever, K. (2010), p. 2028.

167. ANSWER: 1, 2, 3.
Weight reduction decreases stress on the joints. Progressive walking strengthens bone and muscles and helps reduce obesity. Walking should be for a duration that is well tolerated initially, and then walking is gradually increased to 30–60 minutes 5 to 7 days per week. Cold will reduce swelling and inflammation; heat increases circulation to the area and increases comfort. Prolonged standing, kneeling, squatting, and stair climbing should be avoided to protect the knee joint from stress. First-line medications include acetaminophen (Tylenol) or, if that is not effective, a nonsteroidal anti-inflammatory drug (NSAID).

TEST-TAKING TIP: Focus on initial measures to protect the knee joint, reduce pain, and increase activity tolerance.

Content Area: Adult Health; **Category of Health Alteration:** Musculoskeletal Management; **Integrated Processes:** Teaching and Learning; **Client Need:** Physiological Integrity/Physiological Adaptation/Illness Management; **Cognitive Level:** Application; **Reference:** Smeltzer, S., Bare, B., Hinkle, J., & Cheever, K. (2010), pp. 1651–1652; **EBP Reference:** American Academy of Orthopaedic Surgeons (AAOS). (2008). *Treatment of osteoarthritis of the knee (non-arthroplasty).* Rosemont, IL: AAOS. Retrieved from www.guideline.gov/summary/summary.aspx?doc_id=14279&nbr=7155.

168. Which client position should a nurse anticipate when assessing a client in Buck's traction? Place an X on the correct type of traction.

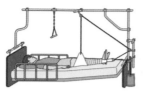

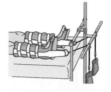

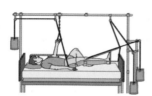

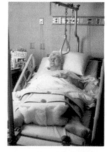

169. Which findings should a nurse associate with the development of compartment syndrome when assessing a client with a cast? **Select all that apply.**

1. Capillary refill time 3 seconds
2. Deep, throbbing, unrelenting pain
3. States feeling "pins and needles" and tingling sensation
4. Nailbeds and fingers swollen and bright pink in appearance
5. States that third finger is touched when pressure is applied to the index finger

168. ANSWER:

In Buck's traction (a type of skin traction), the leg is aligned in a foam boot and traction is applied to the boot frame by the free-hanging weights. The first illustration is Russell's traction, another type of skin traction. The third illustration shows skeletal traction, where traction is applied directly to the bone by use of a metal pin or wire. The fourth illustration shows an abduction wedge to keep the client's legs from internally rotating or crossing. It may be used after a total hip replacement.

TEST-TAKING TIP: If uncertain, look at each illustration carefully. Eliminate the third illustration, because only one leg is in traction. Next, note that the last illustration does not show traction, only a trapeze from a traction bar. Of the two remaining options, consider which would be most effective to stabilize a fracture.

Content Area: Adult Health; **Category of Health Alteration:** Musculoskeletal Management; **Integrated Processes:** Nursing Process Planning; **Client Need:** Physiological Integrity/Reduction of Risk Potential/Therapeutic Procedures; **Cognitive Level:** Application; **Reference:** Smeltzer, S., Bare, B., Hinkle, J., & Cheever, K. (2010), pp. 2032–2033, 2038.

169. ANSWER: 2, 3, 5.

Assessment findings of compartment syndrome include pain, paresthesia (tingling sensation), and loss of ability to discriminate touch (the index finger is the second, not the third finger). Normal capillary refill time is 3 seconds or less. Although edema may obscure the function of arterial pulsation, a pink appearance indicates adequate blood flow. Cyanotic nailbeds would indicate venous congestion and diminished circulation.

TEST-TAKING TIP: Eliminate options with normal findings because compartment syndrome indicates a sudden and severe decrease in blood flow to tissues.

Content Area: Adult Health; **Category of Health Alteration:** Musculoskeletal Management; **Integrated Processes:** Nursing Process Analysis; **Client Need:** Physiological Integrity/Physiological Adaptation/Alterations in Body Systems; **Cognitive Level:** Application; **Reference:** Smeltzer, S., Bare, B., Hinkle, J., & Cheever, K. (2010), pp. 2089–2020.

Test 21: Adult Health: Neurological Management

170. A client with a stroke is diagnosed with left homonymous hemianopsia. Place an X on the box that demonstrates the nurse's interpretation of the visual field defect that this client is experiencing.

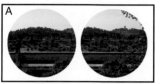

A

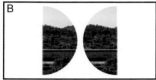

B

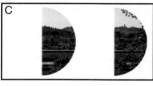

C

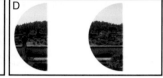

D

171. While sitting on the edge of a bed, a client loses consciousness and experiences a generalized tonic-clonic seizure. Which actions should be taken by a nurse who witnesses the seizure? **Select all that apply.**

1. Guide the client's body to lie in bed, turn the client to the side, and remove objects in the area that could injure the client.
2. Quickly place a padded tongue blade between the client's teeth to prevent tongue laceration.
3. Apply restraints loosely to all four extremities to prevent injury to the client or others.
4. Ascertain if suction equipment is available and request it if it is not in the room.
5. Note the time the seizure started and the progression of events included in the seizure.

170. ANSWER:
Illustration C indicates left homony-
mous hemianopsia, which is blind-
ness in the temporal half of one eye
and the nasal half of the other eye,
occurring on the left side of each
eye. Illustration A is a normal field

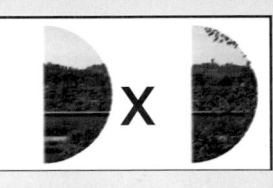

of vision. Illustration B is bi-temporal hemianopsia. With right-sided homonymous hemianopsia the blindness occurs on the right side of each eye as in illustration D.

TEST-TAKING TIP: Key words in the stem include "left homonymous hemi-anopsia" and "visual field defect." Break down the meaning of the term "left homonymous hemianopsia"; "homonymous" means same; "hemi" means half. The left half of the vision field is missing in the view by each eye.

Content Area: Adult Health; **Category of Health Alteration:** Neurological Management; **Integrated Processes:** Nursing Process Analysis; **Client Need:** Physiological Integrity/Reduction of Risk Potential/Potential for Alterations in Body Systems; **Cognitive Level:** Application; **Reference:** Ignatavicius, D., & Workman, M. (2010), p. 1035.

171. ANSWER: 1, 4, 5.
Priority interventions should include preventing injury and maintaining
the airway. Suction equipment should be available to prevent aspiration
if the client has copious secretions or vomits. Because the seizure was
witnessed, the nurse should time and observe the entire seizure. The client should not be restrained, and forcing an object into the client's mouth is likely to cause injury. Tongue lacerations are likely to occur at the beginning of the seizure and would not be prevented.

TEST-TAKING TIP: Key words identify the client is having a tonic-clonic seizure. Consider Maslow's Hierarchy of Needs to address physiological needs of the client and then safety. Use the ABCs (airway, breathing, circulation) to prioritize maintaining the airway. Eliminate options 2 and 3 because these will increase the likelihood of injury to the client.

Content Area: Adult Health; **Category of Health Alteration:** Neurological Management; **Integrated Processes:** Nursing Process Implementation; **Client Need:** Physiological Integrity/Physiological Adaptation/Alterations in Body Systems; **Cognitive Level:** Analysis; **Reference:** Ignatavicius, D., & Workman, M. (2010), p. 955.

172. A nurse assesses a client admitted with a diagnosis of meningitis. Which illustration best describes the nurse's assessment finding that the client has a positive Kernig's sign?

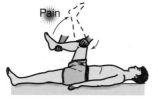

1.

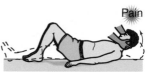

2.

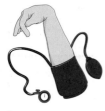

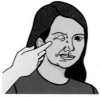

3.

4.

172. ANSWER: 1.
Meningeal irritation from meningitis results in a positive Kernig's sign (illustration 1). To assess for Kernig's sign, the client is recumbent, with the thigh flexed at a right angle to the abdomen and the knee flexed at a 90-degree angle to the thigh. Extension of the lower leg upward causes pain, spasm of the hamstring muscles, and resistance to further leg extension. Meningeal irritation also results in a positive Brudzinski's sign (illustration 2). When the client's neck is flexed, the client experiences neck pain and flexion of the knees and hips. Trousseau's sign (illustration 3) is carpopedal spasm induced when blood flow to the arm is occluded using either a blood pressure cuff or tourniquet. Chvostek's sign (illustration 4) is spasm of the facial muscles produced when the facial nerve in front of the parotid gland and anterior to the ear is tapped. Both Trousseau's sign and Chvostek's sign are suggestive of latent tetany in hypocalcemia.

TEST-TAKING TIP: Focus on the client's diagnosis of meningitis and recall that it produces meningeal irritation. Think about the location of the meninges in the brain and spinal cord. Use this information as a clue to eliminate options 3 and 4. Of the remaining options, use "<u>k</u>ick" (the action seen in the illustration) as a memory cue to "<u>K</u>ernig's sign" and eliminate option 2.

Content Area: Adult Health; **Category of Health Alteration:** Neurological Management; **Integrated Processes:** Nursing Process Assessment; **Client Need:** Physiological Integrity/Physiological Adaptation/Alterations in Body Systems; **Cognitive Level:** Application; **Reference:** Smeltzer, S., Bare, B., Hinkle, J., & Cheever, K. (2010), pp. 1245, 1951.

173. A client had a pituitary tumor surgically removed the previous day. At 1200 hours a nurse documents and reviews the client's electronic medical record (EMR; see exhibit). Based on the information, which should be the nurse's **priority** plan of action?

SCREEN A *Electronically Signed. K.A. Domino, RN*

Date: 1/14/11	0730	0800	1000	1200
Blood pressure (BP)		116/72	98/76	82/48
Pulse		72	90	128
Respirations		28	16	28
Temperature (°F)		99.2°		99.6°
SpO₂		95	98	88
Oxygen		2 L		3 L
Oxygen source		NC		NC
Urine output mL	110	600	700	900
Urine color	Amber	Amber	Clear	Clear
Fingerstick blood glucose (FSG)		150		160

1. Insert a urinary catheter.
2. Recheck the client's blood pressure (BP).
3. Notify the health care provider (HCP).
4. Check to determine if insulin has been ordered.

174. A nurse is teaching a client with Parkinson's disease interventions for dealing with bradykinesia. Which information should the nurse include in the teaching session? **Select all that apply.**

1. Rock back and forth to get going.
2. Maintain a wide-based gait when walking.
3. Pause between every word.
4. Use both hands to accomplish tasks.
5. Visualize your intended movement.

173. ANSWER: 3.

The nurse should notify the HCP because polyuria (large amounts of dilute urine output), hypotension, and tachycardia suggest diabetes insipidus (DI), a complication that can have an abrupt onset within the first few days after neurosurgery. DI is a deficiency of antidiuretic hormone that results in the inability to conserve water. If the client doesn't already have a urinary catheter, the HCP would need to be contacted before one could be placed. The nurse documented the recent BP; retaking another BP would delay contacting the HCP. The fingerstick blood glucose (FSG) is not severely elevated, warranting insulin administration before notifying the HCP.

TEST-TAKING TIP: Think about the complications that can occur after neurosurgery. Note the increasing urine output and the changes in vital signs, which suggest DI.

Content Area: Adult Health; **Category of Health Alteration:** Neurological Management; **Integrated Processes:** Nursing Process Planning; **Client Need:** Physiological Integrity/Reduction of Risk Potential/Changes or Abnormalities in Vital Signs; **Cognitive Level:** Analysis; **Reference:** Black, J., & Hawks, J. (2009), pp. 1059, 1829.

174. ANSWER: 1, 2, 5.

Bradykinesia is slow movements. Measures to enhance movement include rocking back and forth to get started, using a wide-based gate to prevent falling, and visualizing the intended movement. Pausing between words ensures good communication and using both hands will help when tremors interfere with completing tasks; but these do not help with gait.

TEST-TAKING TIP: "Bradykinesia" is slow movements. Use this information to eliminate the options that do not pertain to gait.

Content Area: Adult Health; **Category of Health Alteration:** Neurological Management; **Integrated Processes:** Teaching and Learning; **Client Need:** Physiological Integrity/Physiological Adaptation/Illness Management; **Cognitive Level:** Analysis; **Reference:** Black, J., & Hawks, J. (2009), p. 1906.

Test 22: Adult Health: Perioperative Management

175. A client being admitted as an out-patient for a right total knee replacement confides to a nurse of being fearful because the client had a friend who had eye surgery and they operated on the wrong eye. Which statements should the nurse make in response to the client's concerns? **Select all that apply.**

1. "The nurses and surgeons are so careful that nothing like that has ever happened at this hospital."
2. "You will be asked to mark your own right knee with a permanent marker that this is the correct site to avoid operating on the wrong knee."
3. "Your surgeon will be asked to verify that the right knee is the correct knee and will write his or her initials on your right knee."
4. "An *X* will be made on your left knee so that everyone knows that this knee is the incorrect knee for the knee replacement."
5. "Once you are in the operating room, the nurse will review your chart with you and ask you to identify the knee on which the operation is to be performed."

176. A nurse teaches a client deep breathing and foot exercises to perform postoperatively to prevent complications. The nurse determines that the client can perform the exercises correctly. Place each step in the correct order (1–6) that demonstrates to the nurse that the client is able to complete the exercises correctly, starting with the breathing exercises and ending with the foot exercises.

_____ 1. Pushes the knee down into the mattress

_____ 2. Inhales through the nose until the abdomen distends

_____ 3. Places his or her hands on the abdomen to feel whether the chest rises for full lung expansion

_____ 4. Exhales through pursed lips while contracting the abdominal muscles

_____ 5. Turns the feet in circles and wiggles the toes

_____ 6. Sits upright at the side of the bed or in bed in a semi-Fowler's position

175. ANSWER: 2, 3, 5.
Wrong-site surgeries are avoided by having the client mark the surgical site with a permanent marker, having the surgeon sign the marked site after verifying it as the correct site, and taking a "timeout" in the operating room, which includes corroborating the information and surgical site stated in the client's chart with the client. The Joint Commission does not specify the type of mark, but whatever mark is used, it must be consistently used throughout the facility. Option 1 is giving false reassurances and belittles the client's concerns. Option 4, placing an *X* on the knee not intended to be the site of operation, could result in wrong-site surgery. An *X* is considered ambiguous and should not be used to mark the operative site.

TEST-TAKING TIP: Read each option carefully. Note that options 2 and 4 are opposites. Remember an *X* is ambiguous; thus, eliminate option 4. Consider the false reassurance stated in option 1.

Content Area: Adult Health; **Category of Health Alteration:** Perioperative Management; **Integrated Processes:** Communication and Documentation; **Client Need:** Safe and Effective Care Environment/Safety and Infection Control/Error Prevention; **Cognitive Level:** Analysis; **Reference:** Black, J., & Hawks, J. (2009). pp. 208–210; **EBP Reference:** Institute for Clinical Systems Improvement. (2009). Health Care Protocol: Perioperative Protocol. Retrieved from www.icsi.org/perioperative__protocol__36011/perioperative__protocol.html.

176. ANSWER: 6, 3, 2, 4, 1, 5.
The client should first sit upright at the side of the bed or in a semi-Fowler's position in bed. Next, he or she places his or her hands on the abdomen to feel whether the chest rises for full lung expansion and then inhales through the nose until the abdomen distends. Next, the client exhales through pursed lips while contracting the abdominal muscles. Moving down the body, the client pushes the knee down into the mattress and then turns the feet in circles and wiggles the toes. These exercises are performed to prevent postoperative surgical complications.

TEST-TAKING TIP: Practice deep breathing and foot exercises prior to attempting to place the items in the correct order.

Content Area: Adult Health; **Category of Health Alteration:** Perioperative Management; **Integrated Processes:** Nursing Process Evaluation; **Client Need:** Physiological Integrity/Reduction of Risk Potential/Potential for Complications from Surgical Procedures and Health Alterations; **Cognitive Level:** Application; **Reference:** Black, J., & Hawks, J. (2009). p. 194.

177. A client is to receive one unit of packed red blood cells (480 mL) intravenously (IV) to infuse in 4 hours. How many milliliters per hour (mL/hr) should the nurse set the infusion pump to deliver?

_____ mL/hr (Record your answer as a whole number.)

178. A nurse is planning care for a client following a lumbar laminectomy procedure. In which position should the nurse place the bed for correct positioning of this client following surgery? Place an X on the correct bed position.

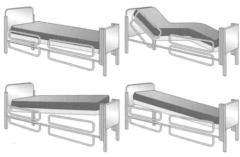

177. ANSWER: 120
Use the formula:

$$\frac{\text{Total mL ordered}}{\text{Total hr ordered}} = \text{mL/hr} \qquad \frac{480 \text{ mL}}{4 \text{ hours}} = 120 \text{ mL/hr}$$

TEST-TAKING TIP: Use a calculation formula to determine the milliliters per hour. Be sure to double-check your answer, especially if it seems unusually large.

Content Area: Adult Health; **Category of Health Alteration:** Perioperative Management; **Integrated Processes:** Nursing Process Implementation; **Client Need:** Physiological Integrity/Pharmacological and Parenteral Therapies/Blood and Blood Products; **Cognitive Level:** Application; **Reference:** Pickar, G., & Abernethy, A. (2008). p. 370.

178. ANSWER:
Following a lumbar laminectomy, the client should be positioned with the bed in a flat position. If the client is positioned supine, a small pillow may be placed under the client's head and the knee elevated slightly to relax the back muscles. If the client turned to a sidelying position, the bed should be flat, 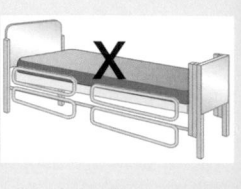 a pillow placed between the client's legs, the client log-rolled, and additional pillows used to support the client's back and upper arm. A contour, Trendelenburg, or reverse Trendelenburg position should be avoided because of spinal instability after surgery.

TEST-TAKING TIP: Apply knowledge of medical terminology: "lumbar" is the lower back, "lamina" is a part of the vertebrae, and "-ectomy" is removal of. Consider the instability of the spine when selecting an option.

Content Area: Adult Health; **Category of Health Alteration:** Perioperative Management; **Integrated Processes:** Nursing Process Planning; **Client Need:** Physiological Integrity/Basic Care and Comfort/Mobility/Immobility; **Cognitive Level:** Application; **Reference:** Smeltzer, S., Bare, B., Hinkle, J., & Cheever, K. (2010). pp. 469–470, 2002.

Test 23: Adult Health: Renal and Urinary Management

179. A nurse is discharging a client following extracorporeal shock water lithrotripsy (ESWL) for treatment of a renal stone. Which instructions should the nurse include in the discharge teaching? **Select all that apply.**

1. Increase your fluid intake.
2. Report blood-tinged urine to the health care provider (HCP).
3. Expect that a bruise may be observed on the treated side of your back.
4. Check your temperature daily and notify the HCP if your temperature is greater than 101°F (38°C).
5. Check your urine for stone fragments and notify the HCP if fragments are passed.

180. A client had a significant amount of blood loss during surgery and was hypotensive upon return to a surgical unit. Which findings should alert a nurse that the client may be experiencing acute renal failure? **Select all that apply.**

1. Urine specific gravity 1.030
2. Urine output 60 mL/hr
3. ECG changes of peaked T waves
4. Urine sodium increased
5. Urine osmolality increased

179. ANSWER: 1, 3, 4.
An increased fluid intake assists in the passage of stone fragments. Usually a bruise will appear where high-energy dry shock waves pass through the skin to fragment the stone. An elevated temperature may indicate the presence of an infection, and the HCP should be notified. Hematuria is expected and should disappear in 4 to 5 days. It is unnecessary to report this to the HCP. Passing stone fragments in the urine is expected after ESWL. These may be passed for 6 weeks to several months after the procedure.

TEST-TAKING TIP: ESWL uses high-energy dry shock waves to fragment stones. Use this information to eliminate options that would be expected after the procedure.

Content Area: Adult Health; **Category of Health Alteration:** Renal and Urinary Management; **Integrated Processes:** Teaching and Learning; **Client Need:** Health Promotion and Maintenance/Self-care; **Cognitive Level:** Analysis; **Reference:** Smeltzer, S., Bare, B., Hinkle, J., & Cheever, K. (2010), pp. 1378–1380.

180. ANSWER: 1, 3, 5.
In prerenal failure from hypoperfusion, the urine specific gravity is increased. Normal urine specific gravity is 1.010–1.025; an increase in specific gravity indicates the urine is more concentrated. The decline in the glomerular filtration rate, oliguria, and anuria can produce hyperkalemia. ECG changes of tall, tented, or peaked T waves suggest hyperkalemia. Urine osmolality increases in prerenal failure. A urine output of 60 mL/hr is adequate. The urine sodium would be decreased and not increased in prerenal failure.

TEST-TAKING TIP: The key phrase is "blood loss during surgery." Select options that pertain to prerenal failure.

Content Area: Adult Health; **Category of Health Alteration:** Renal and Urinary Management; **Integrated Processes:** Nursing Process Evaluation; **Client Need:** Physiological Integrity/Reduction of Risk Potential/Potential for Alterations in Body Systems; **Cognitive Level:** Analysis; **Reference:** Smeltzer, S., Bare, B., Hinkle, J., & Cheever, K. (2010), pp. 1321–1322; **EBP Reference:** Balas, M., Casey, C., & Happ, M. (2008). Comprehensive assessment and management of the critically ill. In E. Capezuti, D. Zwicker, M. Mezey, & T. Fulmer , (eds.), *Evidence-based geriatric nursing protocols for best practice* (3rd ed., pp. 565–593). New York: Springer Publishing Company.

181. A nurse reads that a client has a urostomy from an ileal conduit created during a urinary diversion procedure. In planning care for this client, which illustration should the nurse visualize when thinking about the type of procedure performed and the type of stoma that the nurse should expect when assessing the client?

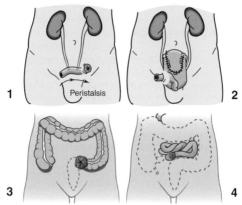

1   Peristalsis

2

3

4

182. A client with chronic glomerulonephritis develops progressive renal failure and has a glomerular filtration rate (GFR) of 45 mL/min. What information should a nurse associate with this problem when reviewing the client's medical record in preparation for care? **Select all that apply.**

1. Hypokalemia
2. Metabolic acidosis
3. Anemia
4. Hypercalcemia
5. Hypoalbuminemia

181. ANSWER: 1.

In an ileal conduit (Illustration 1), the urine is diverted by implanting the ureters into a loop of the ileum and one end is brought out through the abdominal wall. A urostomy bag is used to collect the urine. Illustration 2 is an Indiana pouch, in which the ureters are implanted into a segment of the ileum and cecum and a pouch is created. Urine is drained intermittently by inserting a catheter into the stoma. Illustration 3 is a sigmoid colostomy, in which a segment of the colon is brought outside the abdominal wall. Illustration 4 is an ileostomy in which a segment of the ileum is brought through the abdominal wall.

TEST-TAKING TIP: Note the key words "urinary diversion." Eliminate options that illustrate bowel diversions. Of the remaining two options, eliminate the option with the pouch.

Content Area: Adult Health; **Category of Health Alteration:** Renal and Urinary Management; **Integrated Processes:** Nursing Process Planning; **Client Need:** Physiological Integrity/Physiological Adaptation/Alterations in Body Systems; **Cognitive Level:** Application; **Reference:** Smeltzer, S., Bare, B., Hinkle, J., & Cheever, K. (2010), pp. 1383–1385.

182. ANSWER: 2, 3, 5.

Metabolic acidosis occurs from the decreased acid secretion by the kidney and the inability to regenerate bicarbonate. Anemia is secondary to decreased erythropoietin (production of RBCs). Hypoalbuminemia results from the protein loss through the damaged glomerular membrane and tissue edema. Hyperkalemia (not hypokalemia) occurs due to the decreased potassium excretion, acidosis, catabolism, and excessive potassium intake from food and medications. Hypocalcemia (not hypercalcemia) occurs because calcium binds to phosphorus to compensate for the elevated serum phosphorus levels.

TEST-TAKING TIP: Read each option carefully for "hypo-" and "hyper-" to avoid making an incorrect selection.

Content Area: Adult Health; **Category of Health Alteration:** Renal and Urinary Management; **Integrated Processes:** Nursing Process Assessment; **Client Need:** Physiological Integrity/Physiological Adaptation/Fluid and Electrolyte Imbalances; **Cognitive Level:** Analysis; **Reference:** Smeltzer, S., Bare, B., Hinkle, J., & Cheever, K. (2010), p. 1316.

183. A client had a urinary diversion procedure with creation of an ileal conduit 1 day ago for treatment of bladder cancer. Which actions should be taken by the nurse when caring for this client? **Select all that apply.**

1. Remove the nasogastric tube.
2. Inspect the stoma every 4 hours to ensure that it is red or pink colored.
3. Ask the client to use the patient-controlled analgesia (PCA) prior to transferring to the chair.
4. Encourage the client to deep breath and cough every 1 to 2 hours while awake.
5. Measure the urine output and empty the urine collection bag every 8 hours.

184. A client is taking cyclosporine following a kidney transplant. A nurse is reviewing the client's serum laboratory results. Which finding indicates that the client may be experiencing acute rejection? Place an X on the laboratory value result that suggests acute rejection of the transplanted kidney.

LABORATORY REPORT

Serum Lab Test	Client Result
Creatinine	6.7 mg/dL
White blood cells (WBCs)	4,000/mm³
Platelets	98,000/mm³
Potassium	3.9 mEq/L

183. ANSWER: 2, 3, 4.

A new stoma should be assessed every 4 hours to evaluate the adequacy of its blood supply. The stoma should be red or pink. The use of a PCA prior to activity promotes client comfort and participation in activity. Deep breathing and coughing will prevent atelectasis and pulmonary complications. The NG tube usually remains in place for several days to decompress the gastrointestinal (GI) tract and relieve pressure on the intestinal anastamosis. An ostomy drainage bag is applied over the stoma. Urine output is monitored closely and usually measured every 2 hours.

TEST-TAKING TIP: The client is only 1 day postoperative a urinary diversion. Thinking about the potential complications of ileus and urine leakage should guide you to eliminate options 1 and 5.

Content Area: Adult Health; **Category of Health Alteration:** Renal and Urinary Management; **Integrated Processes:** Nursing Process Implementation; **Client Need:** Physiological Integrity/Physiological Adaptation/Illness Management; **Cognitive Level:** Application; **Reference:** Smeltzer, S., Bare, B., Hinkle, J., & Cheever, K. (2010), pp. 1388–1390.

184. ANSWER:

LABORATORY REPORT

Serum Lab Test	Client Result
Creatinine	6.7 mg/dL [X]

Clients taking cyclosporine may not exhibit the usual signs and symptoms of acute rejection. The only sign may be an asymptomatic rise in the serum creatinine level because the kidney is unable to excrete the by-products of metabolism. Immunosuppression depresses the formation of leukocytes (WBCs) and platelets. The potassium level is normal.

TEST-TAKING TIP: Although a number of laboratory values are abnormal, focus on the laboratory value specific to evaluating renal function.

Content Area: Adult Health; **Category of Health Alteration:** Renal and Urinary Management; **Integrated Processes:** Nursing Process Analysis; **Client Need:** Physiological Integrity/Physiological Adaptation/Unexpected Response to Therapies; **Cognitive Level:** Analysis; **Reference:** Smeltzer, S., Bare, B., Hinkle, J., & Cheever, K. (2010), p. 1353.

185. A female client, who is scheduled for a TRAM (transverse rectus abdominis myocutaneous) flap procedure, questions a nurse about where the tissue will be obtained for her new breast. Place an X within the circled area that the nurse should indicate when answering the client's question.

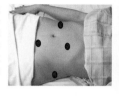

186. A nurse is reviewing the laboratory study results of a client 1 day after a modified radical mastectomy. Based on the results, which action should be the nurse's **priority**?

LABORATORY TEST RESULTS

Test	1 Day Prior to Surgery	4 Hours After Surgery (2100 yesterday)	0600 Today
HGB	14.3 g/dL	11.8 g/dL	8.2 g/dL
HCT	43%	35%	25%
RBC	$4.9 \times 10^8/mm^3$	$4.2 \times 10^8/mm^3$	$3.9 \times 10^8/mm^3$
PLT	$230,000/mm^3$	$161,000/mm^3$	$90,000/mm^3$
WBC	$9,000/mm^3$	$12,000/mm^3$	$14,000/mm^3$

1. Notifying the health care provider (HCP) of the laboratory results
2. Donning gloves and assessing for the source of the blood loss
3. Checking to determine if the client has an antibiotic to be administered
4. Taking the client's vital signs

185. ANSWER:
The TRAM flap procedure involves the use of the client's own tissue. Skin, fat, and muscle with attached blood supply are taken from the lower abdomen to the operative breast area. The abdominal tissue is similar in consistency to the natural breast.

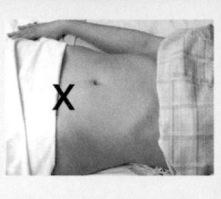

TEST-TAKING TIP: The name of the surgical procedure should provide a hint as to the part of the body used.

Content Area: Adult Health; **Category of Health Alteration:** Reproductive Management; **Integrated Processes:** Teaching and Learning; **Client Need:** Physiological Integrity/Physiological Adaptation/Alterations in Body Systems; **Cognitive Level:** Application; **References:** Ignatavicius, D., & Workman, M. (2010), pp. 1675–1676; Smeltzer, S., Bare, B., Hinkle, J., & Cheever, K. (2010), p. 1498.

186. ANSWER: 2.
The laboratory test results suggest the client is bleeding. The nurse should first assess for the source of the bleeding. The nurse needs additional information before notifying the HCP. Although the white blood cell count (WBC) is elevated and an antibiotic should be prescribed, this is not the priority because a significant amount of blood has been lost. The vital signs will give information about adequate perfusion; however, if the client is bleeding, pressure needs to be applied to staunch the blood flow.

TEST-TAKING TIP: Consider that the laboratory test results suggest that the client is bleeding.

Content Area: Adult Health; **Category of Health Alteration:** Reproductive Management; **Integrated Processes:** Nursing Process Implementation; **Client Need:** Physiological Integrity/Physiological Adaptation/Unexpected Response to Therapies; **Cognitive Level:** Analysis; **Reference:** Black, J., & Hawks, J. (2009), p. 956.

187. A nurse is assessing a client with pelvic inflammatory disease (PID). Which findings should a nurse conclude are consistent with the diagnosis? **Select all that apply.**

1. Presence of a myoma
2. States experiencing dyspareunia
3. Lower abdominal pain
4. Tenderness that occurs after menses
5. Vaginal discharge

188. A nurse is admitting a 56-year-old client who is to have an abdominal hysterectomy for uterine fibroids and polycystic ovaries. When reviewing the list of medications, herbal products, and supplements that the client brought from home, which items on the list should prompt the nurse to question the client about experiencing menopausal symptoms? Place an X on the items that prompted the nurse's questioning.

MEDICATION LIST: JONES, DARLENE

Birthdate: 01-01-1954	Allergies: None
Scheduled	**Last Taken**
Black cohosh 40 mg oral daily	0800 today
Metformin (Fortamet) 500 mg bid	0800 today
Vitamin E 400 international units bid	0800 today
PRN	**Last Taken**
Diphenhydramine (Benadryl) 25 mg oral prn pruritus	1900 two days ago

187. ANSWER: 2, 3, 4, 5.
PID is an inflammatory condition of the pelvic cavity from an infection that may be acute, subacute, recurrent, or chronic. Symptoms usually begin with vaginal discharge, dyspareunia (painful intercourse), lower abdominal pelvic pain, and tenderness that occurs after menses. A myoma is a usually benign fibroid tumor of the uterus arising from the muscle tissue of the uterus.

TEST-TAKING TIP: The key word is "inflammatory." Eliminate option 1 because it is not associated with an inflammatory disorder.

Content Area: Adult Health; **Category of Health Alteration:** Reproductive Management; **Integrated Processes:** Nursing Process Assessment; **Client Need:** Physiological Integrity/Physiological Adaptation/Alterations in Body Systems; **Cognitive Level:** Application; **Reference:** Smeltzer, S., Bare, B., Hinkle, J., & Cheever, K. (2010), pp. 1446, 1453–1454.

188. ANSWER:

Black cohosh 40 mg oral daily	0800 today
Vitamin E 400 international units bid	0800 today

Black cohosh, an herbal product, is commonly used to treat menopausal symptoms. Although the mechanism of action is unclear, research supports that women using black cohosh experience fewer menopausal symptoms. Vitamin E (800 international units) reduces vasomotor symptoms (hot flashes). Metformin, in addition to being an oral antidiabetic agent, lowers testosterone production in a client with polycystic ovary syndrome. A side effect of black cohosh is a rash. Diphenhydramine may have been used to control itching associated with a rash.

TEST-TAKING TIP: If unsure, select the options that include herbal products and oral supplements.

Content Area: Adult Health; **Category of Health Alteration:** Reproductive Management; **Integrated Processes:** Nursing Process Evaluation; **Client Need:** Physiological Integrity/Physiological Adaptation/Alterations in Body Systems; **Cognitive Level:** Analysis; **Reference:** Osborn, S., Wraa, C., & Watson, A. (2010), pp. 1546, 1550, 1552; **EBP Reference:** Dennehy, C. (2006). The use of herbs and dietary supplements in gynecology: An evidence-based review. *Journal of Midwifery and Women's Health, 61*(6), 402–409.

Test 25: Adult Health: Respiratory Management

189. A nurse is performing a physical assessment of a client. Which sound should a nurse expect to hear when auscultating the circled areas indicated in the exhibit?

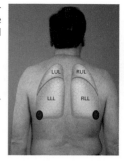

1. Bronchial breath sounds
2. Vesicular breath sounds
3. Popping with long inspiratory phase
4. High-pitched sounds with prolonged inspiratory phase

190. A nurse is preparing to care for a client with chronic obstructive pulmonary disease (COPD). Which interventions should a nurse include when planning the client's care? **Select all that apply.**

1. Teach the client pursed-lip breathing.
2. Teach about the various positions for performing postural drainage.
3. Educate the client on the hazards of tobacco smoking and secondhand smoke.
4. Instruct the client on receiving an annual pneumococcal and influenza vaccine.
5. Determine if vaporization therapy has reduced the client's secretions.

189. ANSWER: 2.
Vesicular sounds should be heard over this area and should be soft and low pitched, like a rustling, from air moving through small airways. They are heard longer during expiration. Bronchial breath sounds are heard lateral to the spine between the third and sixth intercostal spaces. Popping and a long expiratory phase is associated with crackles, and a high-pitched sound indicates wheezing or stridor.

TEST-TAKING TIP: Consider the location of the sound and eliminate the sound heard over larger airways. Then eliminate the two abnormal sounds.

Content Area: Adult Health; **Category of Health Alteration:** Respiratory Management; **Integrated Processes:** Nursing Process Assessment; **Client Need:** Health Promotion and Maintenance/Techniques of Physical Assessment; **Cognitive Level:** Application; **Reference:** Osborn, S., Wraa, C., & Watson, A. (2010), pp. 874–875.

190. ANSWER: 1, 2, 3.
Pursed-lip breathing (controlled breathing) helps to keep the airways open longer to improve ventilation. Postural drainage mobilizes secretions that can obstruct the airways and cause respiratory complications. Smoking causes bronchial constriction and inflammation and increases mucus production. Although pneumococcal and influenza vaccines are recommended, the pneumococcal vaccine is usually administered only once. A second dose is recommended for people 65 years and older who received their first dose when they were younger than 65 and 5 or more years has elapsed since the first dose. The influenza vaccine is administered annually. Although vaporization therapy is used to reduce secretions, this is an evaluation and not an intervention.

TEST-TAKING TIP: Consider the frequency for administering vaccines and then eliminate option 4. Use the nursing process and eliminate any option that is not an intervention but an evaluation, option 5.

Content Area: Adult Health; **Category of Health Alteration:** Respiratory Management; **Integrated Processes:** Nursing Process Planning; **Client Need:** Physiological Integrity/Physiological Adaptation/Illness Management; **Cognitive Level:** Application; **Reference:** Osborn, S., Wraa, C., & Watson, A. (2010), pp. 957–963; **EBP Reference:** Centers for Disease Control and Prevention (2010, March). *Pneumococcal Vaccination.* Retrieved from www.cdc.gov/vaccines/vpd-vac/pneumo/default.htm#vacc.

191. A client experienced a tension pneumothorax. In explaining this to the client, which illustration should a nurse select?

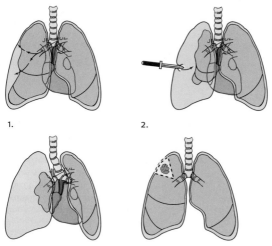

1.

2.

3.

4.

192. A nurse is to administer terbutaline (Brethaire) 250 mcg subcutaneously to a client experiencing acute symptoms associated with chronic obstructive pulmonary disease. The medication label reads 1 mg/mL. How many milliliters (mL) should the nurse administer?

_____ mL (Record your answer to the nearest hundredth.)

191. ANSWER: 3.

A tension pneumothorax occurs from an air leak in the lung or the chest wall on the affected side. The air that enters the pleural space does not exit during expiration and causes an increase in intrapleural pressure. This increased pressure pushes the heart and mediastinal structures to the contralateral side compressing the contralateral lung. The first illustration shows a spontaneous pneumothorax from air entering the pleural space. This can occur from weakened lung tissue or a blisterlike defect in the lung tissue (bullae or blebs). The second illustration is a traumatic pneumothorax in which a penetrating trauma to the chest wall and parietal pleura allows air to enter the pleural space. The fourth illustration shows a segmental resection of the lung in which a portion of the lung tissue is removed.

TEST-TAKING TIP: Examine each illustration closely. If uncertain, select the illustration that would jeopardize oxygen exchange the most.

Content Area: Adult Health; **Category of Health Alteration:** Respiratory Management; **Integrated Processes:** Teaching and Learning; **Client Need:** Physiological Integrity/Physiological Adaptation/Alterations in Body Systems; **Cognitive Level:** Application; **References:** Ignatavicius, D., & Workman, M. (2010), pp. 698–699; Osborn, S., Wraa, C., & Watson, A. (2010), pp. 988–989.

192. ANSWER: 0.25

First, convert milligrams (mg) to micrograms (mcg). 1 mg = 1,000 mcg. Then use the formula for calculating medication dosages.

Formula:

$$\frac{\text{Desired}}{\text{Have}} \times mL = mL/dose$$

$$\frac{250 \text{ mcg}}{1,000 \text{ mcg}} \times 1 \text{ mL} = 0.25 \text{ mL}$$

TEST-TAKING TIP: Remember that 1 mg = 1,000 mcg.

Content Area: Adult Health; **Category of Health Alteration:** Respiratory Management; **Integrated Processes:** Nursing Process Implementation; **Client Need:** Physiological Integrity/Pharmacological and Parenteral Therapies/Dosage Calculation; **Cognitive Level:** Application; **References:** Deglin, J., Vallerand, A., & Sanoski, C. (2011), p. 1197; Osborn, S., Wraa, C., & Watson, A. (2010), p. 957.

193. A client is having respiratory distress related to an anxiety attack. Recent arterial blood gas (ABG) values and a nursing narrative note are provided as illustrated. Based on the information presented, which conclusion about the client should be made by the nurse?

LABORATORY REPORT

Arterial Blood Gas	Result	Normal Range
pH	7.53	7.35–7.45
PaO_2	72	80–100 mm Hg
$PaCO_2$	32	35–45 mm Hg
Bicarbonate (HCO_3)	28	22–26 mEq/L

NURSING NOTE

1900	History of anxiety. Very distraught after cancer diagnosis. Reports restlessness and unease. Provided consolation and support during blood draw and in regards to diagnosis. Will reevaluate after client's visitors leave. N. Bron, RN _____

1. The client is probably overreacting to the situation.
2. The client is probably hyperventilating.
3. The client has acidotic blood.
4. The client is fluid volume depleted.

194. A client is receiving treatment for pleural effusion. Which findings indicate to a nurse that treatment for the pleural effusion has been effective? **Select all that apply.**

1. Lower lung bases dull with percussion.
2. Absence of a pleural friction rub.
3. Severe breathlessness reduced to slight dyspnea.
4. Normal lung sounds auscultated in all lung lobes.
5. Chest x-ray shows blunting of the costophrenic angle.

193. ANSWER: 2.

Clients with anxiety may hyperventilate, causing a "blowing off" of carbon dioxide resulting in a low PaCO$_2$ level and respiratory alkalosis. The arterial blood gas analysis is abnormal, indicating a physiological problem. Merely stating the client is overreacting is an insufficient analysis of the information. The lab results indicate respiratory alkalosis as a result of hyperventilation, not acidosis. No inferences can be made about the client's fluid volume status from the information presented.

TEST-TAKING TIP: Analyze all of the clues provided to determine the best option. Recognize that the ABG results are abnormal so that there is a physiological problem taking place.

Content Area: Adult Health; **Category of Health Alteration:** Respiratory Management; **Integrated Processes:** Nursing Process Analysis; **Client Need:** Physiological Integrity/Reduction of Risk Potential/Laboratory Values; **Cognitive Level:** Analysis; **Reference:** Kee, J. (2009), pp. 66–68.

194. ANSWER: 2, 4.

A pleural effusion is presence of fluid in the pleural space inhibiting full lung expansion. Pleural inflammation can cause a pleural friction rub. The absence of a pleural friction rub and full lung expansion as evidenced by normal lung sounds in all lung lobes are normal findings and indicate treatment is effective. Dullness on percussion indicates the presence of fluid. A reduction of breathlessness shows improvement, but slight dyspnea can occur with fluid accumulation or atelectasis. A blunting of the costophrenic angle as seen on chest x-ray occurs when more than 200–500 mL of fluid is present in the pleural space.

TEST-TAKING TIP: Eliminate options of abnormal findings and any option that shows only a slight improvement.

Content Area: Adult Health; **Category of Health Alteration:** Respiratory Management; **Integrated Processes:** Nursing Process Evaluation; **Client Need:** Physiological Integrity/Reduction of Risk Potential/System Specific Assessments; **Cognitive Level:** Analysis; **Reference:** Osborn, S., Wraa, C., & Watson, A. (2010), pp. 984–985.

Test 26: Adult Health: Vascular Management

195. A nurse is treating clients in a hypertension clinic. Which nursing actions should be initiated to assist the clients who use tobacco to quit and remain tobacco-free? **Select all that apply.**

1. Assess and document smoking status as part of the vital signs assessment with all client visits.
2. Positively reinforce clients who have quit tobacco use and offer assistance to solve problems associated with the decision.
3. Discuss weight gain that may result after the client has quit tobacco use.
4. With clients who have expressed no interest in quitting tobacco use or have relapsed after quitting, offer a motivation to quit tobacco use with each encounter.
5. Encourage participation in a weight loss program for persons who are in a tobacco-use cessation program.

196. A nurse is assessing a client with a diagnosis of left popliteal aneurysm. Identify with an X the area that the nurse should observe and carefully palpate to assess the involved location.

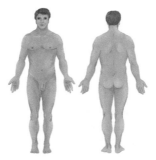

195. ANSWER: 1, 2, 3, 4.
Recommendations for smoking cessation based on evidence include screening all clients for status of tobacco use, offering all clients smoking cessation advice/interventions, and warning that weight gain is likely following cessation. Discussing a weight loss program, if needed, should occur after the client is confident of avoiding relapse.

TEST-TAKING TIP: Read each option carefully. Consider eliminating the one option that is not directly related to smoking cessation.

Content Area: Adult Health; **Category of Health Alteration:** Vascular Management; **Integrated Processes:** Nursing Process Implementation; **Client Need:** Health Promotion and Maintenance/Health Promotion and Disease Prevention; **Cognitive Level:** Analysis; **Reference:** Ignatavicius, D., & Workman, M. (2010), p. 85; **EBP References:** Registered Nurses Association of Ontario (2007). Integrating smoking cessation into daily nursing practice. Retrieved from www.guideline.gov/summary/summary.aspx?doc_id=11503&nbr=005957&string=tobacco+AND+cessation; Rice, V., & Stead, L. (2008). Nursing interventions for smoking cessation. *Cochrane Database of Systematic Reviews*, Issue 1, Art. No.: CD001188. DOI: 10.1002/14651858.CD001188.pub3. Retrieved from www.cochrane.org/reviews/en/ab001188.html.

196. ANSWER:
The left popliteal pulse is assessed in the space behind the left knee, dorsal surface.

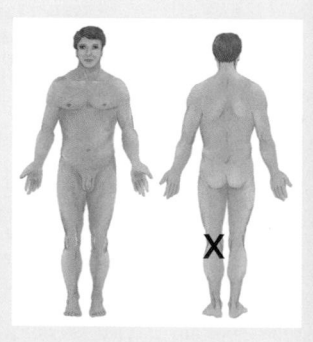

TEST-TAKING TIP: The word "popliteal" is the key word in the stem. Be sure to read the question carefully and only place an X on the left side of the body.

Content Area: Adult Health; **Category of Health Alteration:** Vascular Management; **Integrated Processes:** Nursing Process Assessment; **Client Need:** Physiological Integrity/Physiological Adaptation/Alterations in Body Systems; **Cognitive Level:** Application; **Reference:** Ignatavicius, D., & Workman, M. (2010), pp. 714–718.

197. A nurse assesses a client who presents to a health clinic with an arterial ulcer of the right lower extremity secondary to peripheral arterial disease (PAD). Which findings are consistent with the client's condition? **Select all that apply.**

1. The ulcer is located in the ankle area.
2. The right dorsalis pedis pulse is not palpable, the posterior pulse is weakly palpable.
3. The client guards the ulcer site because of severe pain when the ulcer is touched.
4. The skin around the ulcer has brown discoloration.
5. The client experiences right calf pain after walking a short distance that resolves with rest.

198. A nurse is caring for a 54-year-old female client who had an aortic abdominal aneurysm repaired with a Dacron graft. Which laboratory results should prompt the nurse to consider that the client is experiencing complications following surgery? **Select all that apply.**

SERUM LABORATORY TEST RESULTS

Test	Admit	Day 2	Today (Day 3)
Hgb	9.3 g/dL	12.1 g/dL	11.6 g/dL
Hct	27.9%	36.3%	34.8%
RBC	3.9 m/mm^3	4.2 m/mm^3	3.99 m/mm^3
Plt	260,000/mm^3	361,000/mm^3	320,000/mm^3
WBC	9,000/mm^3	12,000/mm^3	14,000/mm^3
SCr	1.1 mg/dL	2.0 mg/dL	3.1 mg/dL
BUN	31 mg/dL	38 mg/dL	48 mg/dL
Glucose	107 mg/dL	119 mg/dL	130 mg/dL

1. Hemoglobin (Hgb) and hematocrit (Hct)
2. Red blood cells (RBCs) and platelets (Plt)
3. White blood cells (WBCs)
4. Creatinine (SCr) and blood urea nitrogen (BUN)
5. Glucose

197. ANSWER: 2, 3, 5.
In PAD partial or total arterial occlusion deprives the lower extremities of oxygen and nutrients. An unpalpable right dorsalis pedis pulse and a weakly palpable posterior pulse occur due to occlusion. The client initially has severe pain with an arterial ulcer due to impaired blood flow. Intermittent claudication (calf pain after walking a short distance that resolves with rest) also occurs from impaired blood flow. Venous ulcers are commonly found in the ankle area along with brown discoloration or stasis dermatitis. Arterial ulcers often occur on the toes or upper aspect of the foot.

TEST-TAKING TIP: The words "arterial ulcer" are key words in the stem. Think about the effects of decreased peripheral perfusion.

Content Area: Adult Health; **Category of Health Alteration:** Vascular Management; **Integrated Processes:** Nursing Process Analysis; **Client Need:** Physiological Integrity/Physiological Adaptation/Alterations in Body Systems; **Cognitive Level:** Application; **Reference:** Ignatavicius, D., & Workman, M. (2010), pp. 804–805.

198. ANSWER: 3, 4.
The WBCs are increasing, suggesting an infection. The SCr and BUN are elevated indicating renal impairment. The Hgb and Hct were initially low when the client was admitted, increased on day 2, and decreased slightly on day 3. These are expected findings because the client would receive blood replacement during surgery; the decrease on day 3 could be dilutional. The RBCs and Plt are within the normal ranges. Although the glucose level is elevated, this is an expected response with surgical stress and does not suggest a complication.

TEST-TAKING TIP: The key word is "complications." Eliminate the one abnormal laboratory value that is altered with surgical stress. Of the remaining, select the laboratory values that show a progressive increase outside of the normal ranges. Knowing normal laboratory value ranges for these is expected on the NCLEX-RN.

Content Area: Adult Health; **Category of Health Alteration:** Vascular Management; **Integrated Processes:** Nursing Process Evaluation; **Client Need:** Physiological Integrity/Reduction of Risk Potential/Laboratory Values; **Cognitive Level:** Analysis; **Reference:** Osborn, S., Wraa, C., & Watson, A. (2010), pp. 1343–1344.

199. Four clients are admitted to an emergency department at the same time. Prioritize the order in which the nurse should plan to attend to these clients. Place each client in the correct numerical order (1–4).

_____ 1. 37-year-old client who was being treated at home for a deep vein thrombosis who is being admitted with dyspnea.

_____ 2. 45-year-old client admitted with abrupt onset severe, tearing chest pain that radiates to the back.

_____ 3. 76-year-old client who had a right modified radical mastectomy with removal of the lymph nodes who now has 3+ pitting edema and heaviness in the right arm.

_____ 4. 65-year-old client with chronic venous insufficiency admitted because the client has an ankle ulcer with yellow-green drainage and a temperature of 103.7°F (40°C).

200. A nurse is teaching a client with Buerger's disease about self-care management. Which topics should the nurse include in the teaching plan? **Select all that apply.**

1. Smoking cessation
2. Inspecting the extremities for skin breakdown or ulceration
3. Taking aspirin 650 mg twice daily
4. Warming the car before driving in cold weather
5. Increasing potassium in the diet

199. ANSWER: 2, 1, 4, 3.
The 45-year-old client admitted with abrupt onset severe, tearing chest pain that radiates to the back should be attended to first. The client has classic symptoms of aortic dissection, which is a life-threatening condition whereby the intimal layer of the aorta separates, creating a tear in the lumen of the aorta. Next to be seen should be the 37-year-old client who was being treated at home for a deep vein thrombosis who is being admitted with dyspnea. The client may be experiencing a pulmonary embolus. The third client should be the 65-year-old male client with chronic venous insufficiency admitted because an ulcer on his ankle has yellow-green drainage. The drainage suggests an infection. The last client to be attended to is the 76-year-old client who had a right modified radical mastectomy with removal of the lymph nodes who now has 3+ pitting edema and heaviness in the right arm. Although the client has lymphedema, it is not life-threatening and can be treated with limb elevation and a compression garment.

TEST-TAKING TIP: Consider the potential complications that each client could be experiencing. A client with a life-threatening condition should be attended to first. Use the ABCs to establish priority.

Content Area: Adult Health; **Category of Health Alteration:** Vascular Management; **Integrated Processes:** Nursing Process Planning; **Client Need:** Safe and Effective Care Environment/Management of Care/Establishing Priorities; **Cognitive Level:** Analysis; **Reference:** Osborn, S., Wraa, C., & Watson, A. (2010), pp. 1344, 1353, 1355, 1357–1358.

200. ANSWER: 1, 2, 4.
Buerger's disease occurs from an inflammatory response that results in thrombus formation and occlusion of the small vessels in both hands and feet, most commonly from heavy tobacco use. The impaired circulation can lead to skin breakdown and ulceration. Cold environments can cause vasoconstriction, further impairing circulation. Although antiplatelet medication is prescribed, this dose of aspirin is excessive. Increasing potassium will have no effect on Buerger's disease.

TEST-TAKING TIP: Focus on selecting options related to impaired circulation. Eliminate option 3 because the dose is excessive.

Content Area: Adult Health; **Category of Health Alteration:** Vascular Management; **Integrated Processes:** Teaching and Learning; **Client Need:** Health Promotion and Maintenance/Self-care; **Cognitive Level:** Application; **Reference:** Osborn, S., Wraa, C., & Watson, A. (2010), p. 1338.

Test 27: Adult Health: Pharmacological and Parenteral Therapies

201. Cimetidine (Tagamet) is administered to a client with gastro-esophageal reflux disease (GERD). Which findings should lead a nurse to conclude that the client is experiencing side effects from the medication? **Select all that apply.**

1. Pyrosis
2. Impotence
3. Gynecomastia
4. Reduced libido
5. Dyspepsia

202. During an admission assessment to a telemetry unit, a client acknowledges using the herbal supplement valerian. Which follow-up questions by the nurse would be most appropriate? **Select all that apply.**

1. "Have you been having difficulty sleeping or feeling restless?"
2. "How effective has valerian been in relieving your allergy and cold symptoms?"
3. "About how long after taking valerian did you begin experiencing heart palpitations?"
4. "What changes have you noted in your short-term memory since you started using valerian?"
5. "On what areas of your body have you been applying valerian?"

201. ANSWER: 2, 3, 4.
Cimetidine is a histamine H2-receptor-blocking drug that reduces post-prandial daytime and nighttime gastric acid secretion. The side effects of impotence, gynecomastia, and reduced libido occur from the binding of cimetidine to androgen receptors, producing receptor blockage. Pyrosis (retrosternal burning) and dyspepsia are symptoms of GERD and could indicate that the medication is ineffective or the dose is too low.

TEST-TAKING TIP: Eliminate options that are symptoms of GERD to narrow the options to the side effects of the medication.

Content Area: Adult Health; **Category of Health Alteration:** Pharmacological and Parenteral Therapies; **Integrated Processes:** Nursing Process Evaluation; **Client Need:** Physiological Integrity/Pharmacological and Parenteral Therapies/ Adverse Effects/Contraindications/Interactions; **Cognitive Level:** Application; **References:** Ignatavicius, D., & Workman, M. (2010), p. 1244; Spratto, G., & Woods, A. (2010), pp. 338–342.

202. ANSWER: 1, 3.
Valerian is a sedative primarily used to promote sleep or reduce restless-ness. Prolonged use of valerian can cause cardiac abnormalities. Questions about allergy or cold symptoms, memory changes, or topical application of valerian are inappropriate to ask. Either Echinacea or ma huang (ephedra) is used to treat influenza or a common cold. Ginkgo biloba is used to improve memory, sharpen concentration, and promote clear thinking. Topical Echinacea is used to treat wounds, burns, eczema, psoriasis, and herpes simplex infections.

TEST-TAKING TIP: Apply knowledge that valerian promotes sleep to select option 1 and that the client is on a telemetry unit to select option 3.

Content Area: Adult Health; **Category of Health Alteration:** Pharmacological and Parenteral Therapies; **Integrated Processes:** Nursing Process Assessment; **Client Need:** Physiological Integrity/Pharmacological and Parenteral Therapies/ Adverse Effects/Contraindications/Side Effects/Interactions; **Cognitive Level:** Analysis; **Reference:** Lehne, R. (2007), pp. 1238–1244.

203. A nurse is performing admission assessments on clients who visit a health care clinic for the first time. Which client illustrated is most likely to report taking propylthiouracil (PTU) daily?

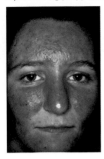

1. Client A

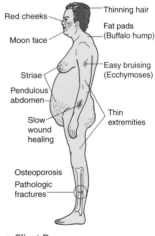

2. Client B

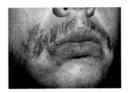

Thinning hair

Red cheeks

Fat pads
(Buffalo hump)

Moon face

Easy bruising
(Ecchymoses)

Striae

Pendulous
abdomen

Slow
wound
healing

Thin
extremities

Osteoporosis
Pathologic
fractures

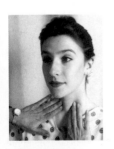

3. Client C

4. Client D

203. ANSWER: 3.
Illustration C shows a woman whose thyroid is being palpated for hyper-thyroidism. Propylthiouracil (PTU) inhibits thyroid hormone synthesis and is used to treat hyperthyroidism or Graves' disease. Illustration A shows a client with lupus erythematosis with the characteristic butterfly rash. Illustration B shows a client with herpes simplex on the face and lips. Illustration D shows a client with Cushing's syndrome, a disorder related to abnormal adrenal function.

TEST-TAKING TIP: Use the process of elimination and knowledge that PTU is used in the treatment of Graves' disease.

Content Area: Adult Health; **Category of Health Alteration:** Pharmacological and Parenteral Therapies; **Integrated Processes:** Nursing Process Assessment; **Client Need:** Physiological Integrity/Pharmacological and Parenteral Therapies/ Expected Actions or Outcomes; **Cognitive Level:** Analysis; **Reference:** Wilson, B., Shannon, M., Shields, K., & Stang, C. (2008), pp. 1294–1296.

204. A nurse is reviewing a client's serum laboratory report. Which finding indicates that the client is receiving a therapeutic dose of heparin?

Serum Laboratory Test	Client's Value	Normal Values
A. Phosphorus	4.0 mg/dL	2.5–4.5 mg/dL
B. Platelets	300,000/mm³	150,000–450,000/mm³
C. PTT	60 sec	25–38 sec
D. PT	22 sec	11–13.5 sec

1. A
2. B
3. C
4. D

205. A client diagnosed with pneumococcal pneumonia is to be discharged from a hospital on levofloxacin (Levaquin) 500 mg daily for 7 days. Which points should a nurse address when teaching the client about the medication? **Select all that apply.**

1. If symptoms do not improve within 3 days, call your health care provider (HCP).
2. If an allergic reaction occurs, notify your HCP, discontinue use, and never take any other medication with a name that ends with "-oxacin."
3. If tendon pain occurs, take a nonsteroidal anti-inflammatory medication (NSAID) such as ibuprofen for pain relief.
4. Avoid sunlight and if unavoidable, wear sunscreen when outdoors.
5. Report tongue discoloration as this may indicate a superinfection.
6. If a sore throat makes swallowing difficult, break the tablets in half and take one half in the morning and the other half in the evening.

204. ANSWER: 3.
A prolonged partial thromboplastin time (PTT) of 60 seconds falls within the therapeutic range of 1.5–2.5 times the control when a client is on heparin. Protime (PT) is used to measure a therapeutic effect of warfarin (Coumadin). Phosphorus and platelets are indicative of other conditions.

TEST-TAKING TIP: Note the key phrase "therapeutic level of heparin" and recall the laboratory results associated with it.

Content Area: Adult Health; **Category of Health Alteration:** Pharmacological and Parenteral Therapies; **Integrated Processes:** Nursing Process Analysis; **Client Need:** Physiological Integrity/Reduction of Risk Potential/Laboratory Values; **Cognitive Level:** Analysis; **Reference:** Wilson, B., Shannon, M., Shields, K., Stang, C. (2008), pp. 730–733.

205. ANSWER: 1, 2, 4, 5.
Lack of symptom improvement could indicate medication resistance to the infection. Medications ending in "-oxacin" are from the fluoroquinolone medication classification, including levofloxacin. An allergy to one medication in the class would pertain to all medications in the same classification. Levofloxacin causes photosensitivity and can result in sunburn. Superinfections can occur when the normal flora is destroyed. If tendon pain occurs, the client should discontinue the medication and notify the HCP. Tendon pain occurs from an adverse reaction to the medication. Taking NSAIDs can increase the risk of central nervous system (CNS) adverse reactions. Levofloxacin is intended for daily dosing every 24 hours. Tablets can be broken in half, but both pieces should be taken at the same time and not at different times of the day.

TEST-TAKING TIP: Look for key words or phrases in each of the options and apply knowledge of levofloxacin to eliminate options. Recall that an adverse effect common to the fluoroquinolone classification of medications is tendon pain.

Content Area: Adult Health; **Category of Health Alteration:** Pharmacological and Parenteral Therapies; **Integrated Processes:** Teaching and Learning; **Client Need:** Physiological Integrity/Pharmacological and Parenteral Therapies/Medication Administration; **Cognitive Level:** Application; **References:** Aschenbrenner, D., & Venable, S. (2009), pp. 807, 812–813; Wilson, B., Shannon, M., Shields, K., & Stang, C. (2008), pp. 872–874.

206. A client admitted with meningitis is requesting medication for a headache rated 10 on a 0–10 numeric scale. While retrieving the medication at 1100 hours, a nurse checks the client's medical record for the vital signs just obtained by a nursing assistant and the client's medication administration record (MAR). Based on the client's chart findings and rated pain level, which action should be taken by the nurse **first**?

VITAL SIGNS

Time	0800	1200
Blood pressure	120/80	150/90
Apical pulse	100	115
Respirations	22	28
Temperature	99.6°F (38°C)	102.6°F (39°C)

MEDICATION ADMINISTRATION RECORD

PRN Medications	0001–0659	0700–1559	1600–2400
Acetaminophen (Tylenol) 325 mg oral 1–2 tabs q4h prn		0700 NNB (1 tab)	
Oxycodone/acetaminophen (Percocet 5/325) oral 1–2 q4h prn			
Morphine sulfate 2–6 mg IM q4h prn			

1. Notify the client's health care provider (HCP).
2. Administer two oral tablets acetaminophen 325 mg.
3. Administer two oral tablets oxycodone/acetaminophen (Percocet 5/325).
4. Administer morphine sulfate 6 mg intramuscularly.

206. ANSWER: 3.
A combination medication is indicated to treat both the client's pain and the elevated temperature. Oxycodone is a narcotic analgesic that binds to opiate receptors in the CNS and is used to treat moderate to severe pain. Acetaminophen inhibits the synthesis of prostaglandins that may serve as mediators of pain and fever, primarily in the CNS, and can be used to augment the oxycodone and reduce the fever. **The elevated vital signs may be a physiological response to pain and fever.** It is premature to notify the HCP. Acetaminophen alone is insufficient to control severe pain. Morphine sulfate, an opioid analgesic, is used to control pain but has no antipyretic properties.

TEST-TAKING TIP: Use the World Health Organization's three-step analgesic ladder to determine the appropriate pain medication for treating moderate to severe pain. Select a medication that also has antipyretic properties.

Content Area: Adult Health; **Category of Health Alteration:** Pharmacological and Parenteral Therapies; **Integrated Processes:** Caring; **Client Need:** Physiological Integrity/Pharmacological and Parenteral Therapies/Pharmacological Pain Management; **Cognitive Level:** Analysis; **Reference:** Aschenbrenner, D., & Venable, S. (2009), pp. 379–381; **EBP Reference:** Institute for Clinical Systems Improvement. (2008). *Assessment and management of acute pain.* Retrieved from www.guideline .gov/summary/summary.aspx?view_id=1&doc_id=12302.

207. A client who underwent chemotherapy and radiation is receiving epoetin alfa (Epogen). Which finding on the client's laboratory report should prompt the nurse to conclude that treatment is effective? Place an X on the laboratory value(s) that indicates treatment is effective.

Serum Laboratory Test	Client's Value	Normal Values
Potassium	4.0 mEq/L	3.5–5.5 mEq/L
Platelets	300,000/mm³	150,000–450,000/mm³
Red blood cells	4.9 m/mm³	4–6 m/mm³
Hemoglobin	13.1 g/dL	12–15 g/dL
Hematocrit	40%	40%–54%
White blood cells	9,000/mm³	3,900–11,900/mm³
Neutrophils	40%	40%–43%

208. A client is to receive methocarbamol (Robaxin) 2 gram in 150 mL D5W intravenously for control of muscle spasms. In order to infuse the medication over 45 minutes using standard tubing, at how many milliliters per hour (mL/hr) should the nurse set the infusion pump to run?

_____ mL/hr (Record your answer as a whole number.)

207. ANSWER:

Red blood cells	4.9 m/mm³ ☒	4–6 m/mm³
Hemoglobin	13.1 g/dL ☒	12–15 g/dL
Hematocrit	40% ☒	40%–54%

Epoetin alfa stimulates red blood cell growth and maturation in the bone marrow. It will elevate the RBC level, thus also increasing hemoglobin and hematocrit levels.

TEST-TAKING TIP: If unsure, consider the kidney's role in synthesizing erythropoietin, which is necessary for red blood cell production.

Content Area: Adult Health; **Category of Health Alteration:** Pharmacological and Parenteral Therapies; **Integrated Processes:** Nursing Process Evaluation; **Client Need:** Physiological Integrity/Pharmacological and Parenteral Therapies/ Expected Actions or Outcomes; **Cognitive Level:** Analysis; **Reference:** Spratto, G., & Woods, A. (2010), pp. 578–583.

208. ANSWER: 200

Use a proportion formula. Multiply the means (inside values) and extremes (outside values) and solve for X.

150 mL : 45 minutes :: X mL : 60 minutes

45 X = 9,000

X = 200 mL

TEST-TAKING TIP: Read the question carefully. It is asking for the milliliters per hour; 1 hour is equivalent to 60 minutes.

Content Area: Adult Health; **Category of Health Alteration:** Pharmacological and Parenteral Therapies; **Integrated Processes:** Nursing Process Planning; **Client Need:** Physiological Integrity/Pharmacological and Parenteral Therapies/Dosage Calculation; **Cognitive Level:** Application; **References:** Aschenbrenner, D., & Venable, S. (2009), p. 230; Pickar, G., & Abernethy, A. (2008), pp. 46, 344.

209. A 22-year-old hospitalized client develops a rash and complains of itching. At 1600 hours, a nurse reviews the client's medication administration record (MAR). Based on the MAR, which action should be taken by the nurse? **Select all that apply.**

MEDICATION ADMINISTRATION RECORD   **DATE: TODAY**

Client Name: Account Number: Allergies: Cefdinir
Date of Birth: 23456   (Omnicef)
  01-01-1989   Weight: 75 kg   Dx: Sepsis

Scheduled Medications	2400–0759	0800–1559	1600–2359
Piperacillin/tazobactam (Zosyn) 3.375 g IV q6h (give over 90 min)	0200 NSN	0800 DSN 1300 DSN	
Furosemide (Lasix) 40 mg IV now		1530 DSN	
Lactobacillus acidophilus (Intestinex) 1 tab per feeding tube daily		0800 DSN	

PRN Medications	2400–0759	0800–1559	1600–2359
Acetaminophen (Tylenol) 325 mg rectal q4–6h prn temp			
Diphenhydramine (Benadryl) 12.5–25 mg IV prn pruritus			
Hydromorphone (Dilaudid) 1.5 mg q3h prn pain	0145 NSN 0630 NSN	0945 DSN 1515 DSN	
Naloxone (Narcan) 0.1 mg prn opioid reversal			

Sig: Night Shift Nurse, RN/NSN   Day Shift Nurse, RN/DSN

1. Turn off the infusion pump to interrupt infusing the rest of the current Zosyn dose.
2. Notify the health care provider (HCP) of the rash and itching.
3. Administer diphenhydramine (Benadryl).
4. Administer naloxone (Narcan).
5. Question if hydromorphone or furosemide (Lasix) could be the cause of the rash because these were recently administered.
6. Question if the *Lactobacillus acidophilus* could initiate the reaction.

209. ANSWER: 2, 3, 5.
A rash and itching suggests an allergic reaction, and diphenhydramine should be administered as the first action. The client already has one medication allergy. Antibiotics are well-known for causing allergic reactions. The HCP should be notified to evaluate the client's symptoms and to review medications. Diphenhydramine is an antihistamine that will control itching. All medications, including furosemide and hydromorphone, should be reviewed to determine the cause. There is no need to turn off the infusion pump for the Zosyn; the dose should be infused by 1430; it is now 1600. Naloxone is an opioid antagonist and is administered for respiratory depression not pruritus. *Lactobacillus acidophilus* is used to replace normal bacterial flora destroyed by antibiotics and to prevent or treat diarrhea or a secondary yeast infection.

TEST-TAKING TIP: After assessment, treat the client with medications already included on the client's MAR, examine the medications being administered, and then notify the HCP.

Content Area: Adult Health; **Category of Health Alteration:** Pharmacological and Parenteral Therapies; **Integrated Processes:** Nursing Process Implementation; **Client Need:** Physiological Integrity/Pharmacological and Parenteral Therapies/ Adverse Effects/Contraindications/Interactions; **Cognitive Level:** Analysis; **References:** Deglin, J., & Vallerand, A. (2011, pp. 450, 620, 761, 898); Osborn, S., Wraa, C., & Watson, A. (2010), pp. 890, 1972–1973.

210. A client is receiving a continuous insulin intravenous infusion to maintain a blood glucose level between 80 and 120 mg/dL. In addition to monitoring hourly glucose levels, for which signs of hypoglycemia should the nurse monitor the client? **Select all that apply.**

1. Anxiety
2. Loss of consciousness
3. Warm, flushed skin
4. Confusion
5. Seizures

211. A nurse is removing a central venous catheter (CVC) from a client's subclavian vein. Which actions should be taken by the nurse to prevent an air embolus from occurring during removal of the CVC? **Select all that apply.**

1. Administer a prophylactic dose of lidocaine intravenously.
2. Place the client in a recumbent position.
3. Instruct the client to bear down during removal of the catheter (Valsalva's maneuver).
4. Instruct the client to cough frequently during the procedure.
5. Position the client's head so that it is turning away from the insertion site.

210. ANSWER: 1, 2, 4, 5.
Hypoglycemia or low blood glucose levels affect brain function because the brain cells require a constant source of glucose to function properly. Anxiety, loss of consciousness, confusion, and seizures are all symptoms of impaired cerebral functioning associated with hypoglycemia. Warm flushed skin is associated with hyperglycemia.

TEST-TAKING TIP: Focus on the issue of the question, the neurological symptoms associated with hypoglycemia. Consider the symptoms that revolve around proper brain function. Eliminate an option associated with hyperglycemia.

Content Area: Adult Health; **Category of Health Alteration:** Pharmacological and Parenteral Therapies; **Integrated Processes:** Nursing Process Assessment; **Client Need:** Physiological Integrity/Pharmacological and Parenteral Therapies/Adverse Effects/Contraindications/Interactions; **Cognitive Level:** Application; **Reference:** Smeltzer, S., Bare, B., Hinkle, J., & Cheever, K. (2010), pp. 1227–1229.

211. ANSWER: 2, 3.
Insertion or removal of a central line provides an opportunity for air to enter the client's circulation. A recumbent position and the Valsalva's maneuver increase intrathoracic pressure and pressure in the central veins, thus reducing the risk. Intravenous lidocaine should be available in the event the client has dysrhythmias from the removal, but a prophylactic dose is not recommended nor would it prevent air emboli. Frequent coughing during the procedure increases the risk of air embolus. Although turning the client's head away will make it easier to remove the catheter and decrease the risk of infection, it has no effect on preventing air embolism.

TEST-TAKING TIP: Select options that will increase intrathoracic pressure. Focus on preventing air embolism and not infection.

Content Area: Adult Health; **Category of Health Alteration:** Pharmacological and Parenteral Therapies; **Integrated Processes:** Nursing Process Implementation; **Client Need:** Physiological Integrity/Pharmacological and Parenteral Therapies/ Central Venous Access Devices; **Cognitive Level:** Analysis; **Reference:** Osborn, S., Wraa, C., & Watson, A. (2010), p. 515; **EBP Reference:** Infusion Nurses Society. (2006). Infusion Nursing Standards of Practice. *Journal of Infusion Nursing,* 29(1 Suppl), S1–S92.

Tab 5

Physiological Integrity | Child Health

Test 28: Child Health: Growth and Development

212. A nurse is evaluating achievement of fine motor developmental milestones for four children. Which child should the nurse determine has **excelled** in the developmental milestones for the child's age?

12-Month-Old Infant	2-Year-Old Toddler	4-Year-Old Preschooler	8-Year-Old School-Age Child
Uses pincer grasp	Builds tower of 12 cubes	Moves around in a balanced fashion	Prints; writes some letters
Releases and rescues an object	Uses fork, spoon, and knife with supervision	Draws stick figure with six parts	Good eye-hand coordination
Randomly turns pages in a book	Independent toileting	Ties shoelaces	Plays a video game
Feeds self finger foods	Copies a circle	Prints letters	Uses scissors; makes a simple craft

1. 12-month-old infant
2. 2-year-old toddler
3. 4-year-old preschooler
4. 8-year-old school-age child

213. A 7-year-old has encopresis. Which questions would be most important for the nurse to ask the child's parents? **Select all that apply.**

1. "Does your child usually wet the bed at night when at home?"
2. "Are your child's stools large and/or hard?"
3. "Has your child had liquid stools lately?"
4. "Have you noticed that your child has stained underwear?"
5. "Does your child show signs of trying to retain stool, such as grimacing and shifting his or her position?"

212. ANSWER: 2.
A toddler 1–3 years is able to copy a circle. The remaining fine motor behaviors of the 2-year-old toddler indicate that the child is achieving fine motor developmental milestones of a preschooler 3–6 years. The fine motor behaviors of the 12-month-old infant, the 4-year-old preschooler, and the 8-year-old child are age appropriate.

TEST-TAKING TIP: The key word is "excelled." If unsure, think about how many toddlers are independent at toileting at 2 years of age.

Content Area: Child Health; **Category of Health Alteration:** Growth and Development; **Integrated Processes:** Nursing Process Evaluation; **Client Need:** Health Promotion and Maintenance/Aging Process; **Cognitive Level:** Analysis; **Reference:** Ward, S., & Hisley, S. (2009), pp. 668–669.

213. ANSWER: 2, 3, 4, 5.
Encopresis is stool incontinence usually beyond the age of 4 when children should normally be able to control their bowels. Large and/or hard stools can occur due to constipation. If the rectum is impacted with hard stool, semiformed or liquid stool from higher in the intestines may leak around the impacted stool and pass through the rectum causing soiling. Signs of encopresis include evidence of attempts to retain stool. Bedwetting (enuresis) is not associated with encopresis.

TEST-TAKING TIP: If unsure of the term "encopresis," note that all options except one pertain to the bowel.

Content Area: Child Health; **Category of Health Alteration:** Growth and Development; **Integrated Processes:** Nursing Process Assessment; **Client Need:** Physiological Integrity/Reduction of Risk Potential/System Specific Assessments; **Cognitive Level:** Application; **Reference:** Ward, S., & Hisley, S. (2009), p. 805.

214. A school nurse is developing a program to address violence in the schools for children in a middle school. Which points are important for the nurse to consider when planning this project? **Select all that apply.**

1. Some students may not have parenteral role models to assist them to identify alternatives to violent behavior.
2. Measures for adolescents to use less violent means to express themselves should be identified.
3. A peer support program should be suggested because these have been successful for curbing school violence.
4. Bullying is a normal developmental response among teenagers and need not be addressed.
5. Therapeutic counselors should be available in case a student needs follow-up after the presentation.

215. A nurse is monitoring for **untoward** changes in an adolescent's body image and self-esteem. Which statements should be the basis for the nurse's concern? **Select all that apply.**

1. Body changes create feelings of confusion due to a loss of security with a familiar body.
2. Body changes create a need for adolescents to compare their bodies to others.
3. Body changes create an overmagnification of small defects.
4. Body changes create feelings of competence.
5. Body changes create a need for adolescents to be different from their peers.

214. ANSWER: 1, 2, 3, 5.
Many students may not have role models to help them identify alternatives to violent behaviors. Peers may be helpful in this presentation because peers are important to adolescents, and many times they listen to peers rather than adults. It is always important to be prepared and have follow-up opportunities for the client if needed. Bullying can be a very serious form of violence and is not a normal developmental response. It should be addressed.

TEST-TAKING TIP: Awareness of ways to interact with adolescents is helpful.

Content Area: Child Health; **Category of Health Alteration:** Growth and Development; **Integrated Processes:** Teaching and Learning; **Client Need:** Health Promotion and Maintenance/Health Promotion and Disease Prevention; **Cognitive Level:** Application; **Reference:** Ball, J., & Bindler, R. (2008), pp. 232–240.

215. ANSWER: 1, 2, 3.
There is a tremendous feeling of confusion as teenagers experience hormonal changes and changes to their bodies. There may be comparison of their bodies to other bodies as they go through these changes. Many small defects can seem significant to the adolescent. Body changes during adolescence create feelings of inadequacy, not competence. Adolescents seek to be like their peers not different from them.

TEST-TAKING TIP: Eliminate any options with a statement that contains words that are opposite of what is expected. The key word is "untoward."

Content Area: Child Health; **Category of Health Alteration:** Growth and Development; **Integrated Processes:** Nursing Process Assessment; **Client Need:** Health Promotion and Maintenance/Developmental Stages and Transitions; **Cognitive Level:** Analysis; **Reference:** Perry, S., Hockenberry, M., Lowdermilk, D., & Wilson, D. (2010), pp. 1105–1122.

Test 29: Child Health: Cardiovascular Management

216. A nurse is managing care for a pediatric client diagnosed with heart failure secondary to hypertrophic cardiomyopathy (HC). In doing so, the nurse educates the client and parents on the known factors related to this condition. Which factors should the nurse include in this education? **Select all that apply.**

1. HC is a genetic abnormality.
2. HC follows an autosomal dominant inheritance pattern.
3. HC is the least common genetically transmitted cardiovascular disease.
4. The clinical symptoms of HC usually first appear during infancy.
5. Acute care therapy is directed at controlling the heart failure with bedrest, fluid restriction, and pharmacological agents.
6. If the child fails to respond to medical therapy, the prognosis is poor without a heart transplant.

217. A child is diagnosed with pulmonary stenosis. When teaching the parents about the child's condition, the nurse uses a heart illustration. Which location should the nurse show the parents as the affected area? Place an X on the affected area.

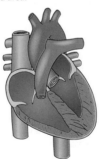

216. ANSWER: 1, 2, 5, 6.

HC follows an autosomal dominant pattern. Symptoms include angina chest pain, dysrhythmias, and syncope. The focus of care is on bedrest to conserve energy, fluid restriction to decrease volume overload, and pharmacological agents to decrease the cardiac load, improve myocardial contractility, and decrease afterload. Heart transplant is an option if the child fails to respond to therapy, but sudden death is possible. HC is the most (not least) common genetically transmitted cardiovascular disease. Symptoms usually appear in the school-age years or adolescence, not during infancy. Presentation in infancy carries a poor prognosis.

TEST-TAKING TIP: The words "hypertrophic cardiomyopathy" are the key words in the stem. If unfamiliar with the condition, apply knowledge of medical terminology. Recall that hypertrophic is increased number of cells, "cardio-" refers to heart, "myo-" refers to muscle, and "pathos-" means disease. Think about a heart that would have impaired filling and ejection because of a decreased size of the chambers. Consider also that the child has one mutant gene and one normal gene. With these in mind, review each of the options.

Content Area: Child Health; **Category of Health Alteration**: Cardiovascular Management; **Integrated Processes:** Teaching and Learning; **Client Need:** Physiological Integrity/Physiological Adaptation/Alterations in Body Systems; **Cognitive Level:** Application; **Reference:** Pillitteri, A. (2010), pp. 1224–1225.

217. ANSWER:

Pulmonary stenosis is a malformation of the pulmonary artery or pulmonic valve. Blood flows from the right ventricle through the pulmonic valve and the pulmonary artery.

TEST-TAKING TIP: Examine the illustration closely to observe the narrowing of the pulmonary artery.

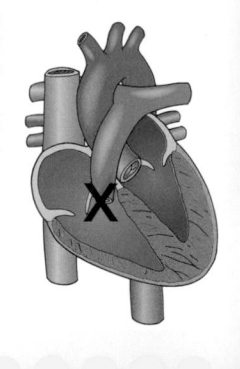

Content Area: Child Health; **Category of Health Alteration:** Cardiovascular Management; **Integrated Processes:** Teaching and Learning; **Client Need:** Physiological Integrity/Physiological Adaptation/ Alterations in Body Systems; **Cognitive Level:** Application; **Reference:** Ward, S., & Hisley, S. (2009), p. 861.

218. A nurse is managing the care of a newborn diagnosed with patent ductus arteriosus (PDA). Which management strategies should the nurse question? **Select all that apply.**

1. Providing respiratory support
2. Administering indomethacin (Indocin)
3. Administering aspirin
4. Regulating fluid intake
5. Preparing for a balloon angioplasty and stent placement
6. Administering ibuprofen (Motrin) intravenously

219. An infant weighing 11 kg has surgery to close an atrial septal defect. The surgeon has written to be notified if the chest tube drainage exceeds 3 mL/kg per hour for 3 consecutive hours. What total amount for the 3 hours should a nurse calculate as the maximum amount of drainage from the infant's chest tube before notifying the surgeon?

_____ mL (Record your answer as a whole number.)

218. ANSWER: 3, 5.
The nurse should question aspirin administration and preparing for a balloon angioplasty and stent placement. The ductus arteriosus is an accessory fetal structure that connects the pulmonary artery to the aorta and begins to close at birth with the first breath. Complete closure usually occurs by 3 months of age. The ductus arteriosus remains open in fetal life due to stimulation by prostaglandins, particularly prostaglandin E (PGE). Prostaglandin inhibitors, such as ibuprofen and indomethacin encourage duct closure. Aspirin is not a prostaglandin inhibitor. A balloon angioplasty and stent placement is a nonsurgical treatment for older infants and adolescents with coarctation of the aorta. Respiratory support due to poor cardiac function and careful fluid regulation to prevent volume overload are other management strategies. Intravenous ibuprofen has been found to be effective in closing a patent ductus arteriosus if it is administered in the first 10–14 days of life.

TEST-TAKING TIP: Select the option that would not be considered a management strategy. Recall that prostaglandin inhibitors are used to encourage closure of the ductus arteriosus.

Content Area: Child Health; **Category of Health Alteration**: Cardiovascular Management; **Integrated Processes:** Nursing Process Implementation; **Client Need:** Physiological Integrity/Physiological Adaptation/Illness Management; **Cognitive Level:** Analysis; **Reference:** Ward, S., & Hisley, S. (2009). pp. 860–862; **EBP Reference:** Ohlsson, A., Walia, R., & Shah, S. (2010). Ibuprofen for the treatment of patent ductus arteriosus in preterm and/or low birth weight infants. *Cochrane Database Systematic Reviews,* Issue 4, Art. No.: CD003481. DOI: 10.1002/14651858. CD003481.pub4. Retrieved from www2.cochrane.org/reviews/en/ab003481.html.

219. ANSWER: 99
The infant weighs 3 kg. Multiple 3 mL × 11 kg = 33 mL/hr. In 3 hours, the drainage should not exceed 99 mL (33 mL × 3 hr = 99 mL/3 hr).

TEST-TAKING TIP: Carefully read the situation. Be sure to determine the amount for 3 hours.

Content Area: Child Health; **Category of Health Alteration:** Cardiovascular Management; **Integrated Processes:** Nursing Process Implementation; **Client Need:** Physiological Integrity/Reduction of Risk Potential/Potential for Complications from Surgical Procedures and Health Alterations; **Cognitive Level:** Application; **Reference:** Ward, S., & Hisley, S. (2009). p. 859.

220. A nurse is receiving a shift report for a pediatric client with rheumatic fever. Which manifestations related to this condition should the nurse prepare to address when caring for this client? **Select all that apply**.

1. Systolic murmur
2. Erythema marginatum
3. Dysfunctional speech
4. Hypothermia
5. Polyarthritis
6. Sebaceous cysts

220. ANSWER: 1, 2, 3, 5.
**A systolic murmur occurs from mitral insufficiency. Erythema margina-
tum, a macular rash found predominantly on the trunk, develops secondary to the inflammatory response. Chorea, sudden involuntary movement
of the limbs, and dysfunctional speech from chorea are due to inflammation of the basal ganglia. Polyarthritis (tender swollen large joints) occur
from the autoimmune response.** Low-grade fever often spiking in the
late afternoon (not hypothermia) reflects an inflammatory process.
Subcutaneous nodules and not sebaceous cysts occur from an autoimmune response. Sebaceous cysts are bumps just beneath the skin that are
filled with an oily, white, semisolid material. They often arise from swollen
hair follicles.

TEST-TAKING TIP: The words "rheumatic fever" and "manifestations"
are the key words in the stem. Recall that rheumatic fever initiates an
autoimmune response.

Content Area: Child Health; **Category of Health Alteration**: Cardiovascular
Management; **Client Need:** Physiological Integrity/Reduction of Risk Potential/
System Specific Assessments; **Cognitive Level:** Application; **Reference:** Ball, J., &
Bindler, R. (2008), pp. 778–779.

Test 30: Child Health: Endocrine Management

221. A nurse is teaching the parents of a 5-year-old child newly diagnosed with type 1 diabetes mellitus (type 1 DM) who is beyond the honeymoon phase of DM. In teaching the parents, which illustration should the nurse select to show the pathophysiology specific to type 1 DM at this stage? Place an X on the illustration that the nurse should select.

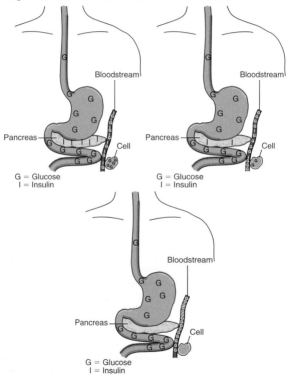

221. ANSWER:

The honeymoon phase is the period during new-onset diabetes when the child has some residual beta-cell function. In type 1 DM, after the honeymoon phase the pancreas is unable to produce insulin due to destruction of the beta cells in the islets of Langerhans. Without insulin, glucose is unable to enter the cells, thus causing hyperglycemia. Illustration 1 shows normal anatomy and physiology. Illustration 2 shows type 2 DM in which a small amount of insulin is produced.

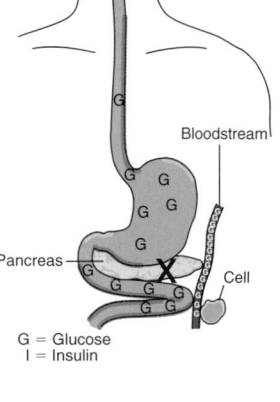

TEST-TAKING TIP: Remember that in type 1 DM there is a failure to produce insulin.

Content Area: Child Health; **Category of Health Alteration:** Endocrine Management; **Integrated Processes:** Teaching and Learning; **Client Need:** Physiological Integrity/Physiological Adaptation/Pathophysiology; **Cognitive Level:** Application; **Reference:** Ball, J., & Bindler, R. (2008). pp. 1223–1225, 1231.

222. An adolescent with type 1 diabetes mellitus (DM) has signed up for participation in the middle school's football program. Which actions should a school nurse take with the football coach to ensure the child's safety during practice sessions and games? **Select all that apply.**

1. Address the importance of monitoring the child's hydration status.
2. Discuss how the ambient temperature of the playing field can affect hydration and blood glucose levels.
3. Identify whether the coach knows how to monitor a blood glucose level.
4. Ensure that the coach determines the type and units of insulin the child has taken that day.
5. Inform the coach to ask the child regarding the composition of the child's previous meal.
6. Tell the coach that the child should not participate because of the possibility of receiving skin lacerations and other injuries on the playing field.

223. A child is experiencing signs of a hypoglycemic episode. What is the correct sequence of the nurse's actions? Place each action in the correct numerical order (1–7).

_____ 1. Wait 15 minutes and check the blood glucose level a second time.

_____ 2. If the blood glucose level is 70 mg/dL or less, give 15 gm of rapid-acting glucose, such as ½ cup fruit juice.

_____ 3. Recheck the blood glucose level for a third time in another 15 minutes.

_____ 4. Obtain a fingerstick blood glucose reading.

_____ 5. Assess for signs of pallor, sweating, tremors, irritability, or an altered mental status.

_____ 6. Repeat the rapid-acting glucose if the blood glucose level is 70 mg/dL or less.

_____ 7. Once the blood sugar has returned to at least 80 mg/dL, give a more substantial snack such as cheese and crackers.

222. ANSWER: 1, 2, 3, 4, 5.
The coach should be able to monitor the child's hydration status, be cognizant of environmental factors that can affect glucose metabolism, be able to check a blood glucose level if needed, and ask the child about the insulin taken and foods eaten to ensure the safety of the child with type 1 DM. The child and coach should also carry a quick source of carbohydrates to treat hypoglycemia. Having type 1 DM does not prevent the child from participating in sports. Precautions should be taken to prevent injuries.

TEST-TAKING TIP: Apply knowledge of glucose-regulating mechanisms and side effects of type 1 DM. Eliminate the one option that is absolute.

Content area: Child Health; **Category of Health Alteration:** Endocrine Management; **Integrated Processes:** Communication and Documentation; **Client Need:** Physiological Integrity/Reduction of Risk Potential/Potential for Alterations in Body Systems; **Cognitive Level:** Application; **Reference:** Ball, J., & Bindler, R. (2008), pp. 1221–1240.

223. ANSWER: 5, 4, 2, 1, 6, 3, 7.
First, assess for signs of pallor, sweating, tremors, irritability, or an altered mental status. Next, obtain a fingerstick blood glucose level. If the blood glucose level is 70 mg/dL or less, give 15 gm of rapid-acting glucose, such as ½ cup fruit juice. Wait 15 minutes and recheck the blood glucose level. Repeat the rapid-acting glucose if the blood glucose level is 70 mg/dL or less. Recheck the blood glucose level in another 15 minutes. Once the blood sugar has returned to at least 80 mg/dL, give a more substantial snack such as cheese and crackers.

TEST-TAKING TIP: Use the nursing process. First select assessment options, then implementation, and then evaluation.

Content Area: Child Health; **Category of Health Alteration:** Endocrine Management; **Integrated Processes:** Nursing Process Implementation; **Client Need:** Physiological Integrity/Reduction of Risk Potential/Potential for Complications from Surgical Procedures and Health Alterations; **Cognitive Level:** Application; **References:** Ball, J., & Bindler, R. (2008), p. 1240; Ward, S., & Hisley, S. (2009), p. 911.

224. A 12-year-old client is preparing to administer a bolus dose of aspart insulin via an insulin pump after eating a meal. A nurse is evaluating if the child is able to calculate the correct amount of insulin. The child is to receive 2 units per 1 carbohydrate choice (1 CHO) eaten. The child ate 100% of the meal in the menu illustrated. If correctly performed by the client, the nurse should observe the child setting the insulin pump to deliver a bolus dose of how many units of aspart insulin?

_____ units (Record your answer as a whole number.)

MENU
Milk 240 mL (1 CHO)
Toast 2 slices (1 CHO per slice)
Butter
Juice 120 mL (1 CHO)
Scrambled eggs
Sausage link

---

225. A 12-year-old client is taking methimazole (Tapazole) and propranolol (Inderal) to treat Graves' disease. The client abruptly discontinues taking the medications and is admitted to an emergency department (ED) 1 week later. Which findings should the nurse expect based on the client's admitting information? **Select all that apply.**

1. Bradycardia
2. Palpitations
3. Muscle weakness
4. Hypotension
5. Tremors

224. ANSWER: 8

Milk is 1 CHO, toast is 2 CHO, and juice is 1 CHO, for a total of 4 CHO. Multiply times 2 units for a total of 8 units.

TEST-TAKING TIP: Carefully read the menu to avoid making an error with the toast.

Content Area: Child Health; **Category of Health Alteration:** Endocrine Management; **Integrated Processes:** Nursing Process Evaluation; **Client Need:** Physiological Integrity/Pharmacological and Parenteral Therapies/Dosage Calculation; **Cognitive Level:** Analysis; **Reference:** Ball, J., & Bindler, R. (2008), pp. 108, 1236–1237.

225. ANSWER: 2, 3, 5.

Because methimazole is given to inhibit thyroid hormone secretion, discontinuing this medication results in excessive levels of circulating thyroid hormones. The client should be assessed for thyrotoxicosis. Signs and symptoms include palpitations, muscle weakness, and tremors. Propranolol, a beta-blocking agent, blocks the action of thyroid hormone on the body thus relieving tachycardia, hypertension, restlessness, and tremors. Discontinuing propranolol results in a resumption of these symptoms. Tachycardia (not bradycardia) and hypertension (not hypotension) would be expected.

TEST-TAKING TIP: Graves' disease results in the oversecretion of thyroid hormone producing hyperthyroidism. A nurse working in the ED should monitor for complications related to hyperthyroidism because the client discontinued taking medications.

Content Area: Child Health; **Category of Health Alteration:** Endocrine Management; **Integrated Processes:** Nursing Process Assessment; **Client Need:** Physiological Integrity/Physiological Adaptation/Unexpected Response to Therapies; **Cognitive Level:** Application; **References:** Ball, J., & Bindler, R. (2008), pp. 1214–1215; Ward, S., & Hisley, S. (2009), p. 897.

Test 31: Child Health: Gastrointestinal Management

226. A nurse is caring for a 10-month-old infant who has intermittent pain that initially starts as sudden, intense pain causing the infant's legs to be drawn up to the abdomen followed by vomiting. After the peristaltic wave passes, the discomfort passes. It has been recurring for the past 12 hours, and now the infant has bloody stools that are "currant jelly–like" in appearance and a rigid, distended abdomen. Emergency surgery is scheduled for an exploratory laparotomy for possible intussusception. Which picture best illustrates a nurse's critical thinking about intussusception as the likely cause of the infant's symptoms and need for surgery?

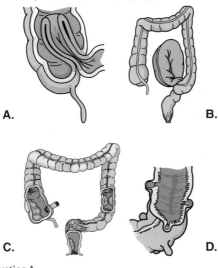

A.

B.

C.

D.

1. Illustration A
2. Illustration B
3. Illustration C
4. Illustration D

226. ANSWER: 1.

Illustration A shows intussusception where a distal segment of the bowel has invaginated into the cecum. Initial intense pain that passes when the peristaltic wave passes, vomiting, and "currant jelly" stools are characteristic symptoms of intussusception. It occurs more commonly in the second half of the first year of life. Illustration B shows a volvulus, bowel twisting and dilated. The twist obstructs the passage of stools, so there would not be currant jelly stools with a volvulus. Usually, a volvulus occurs during the first 6 months of life. Illustration C shows tumors within different sections of the colon; tumors are rare in infants. Illustration D shows diverticuli along the bowel segments. Meckel's diverticulum is the remains of a small pouch of a duct off the ileum. It is the most common congenital malformation of the GI tract, with most symptomatic cases seen in childhood. Currant jelly–like stools can occur with Meckel's diverticulum.

TEST-TAKING TIP: Focus on the infant's signs and symptoms and the medical diagnosis. As a memory aid for intussusception remember "into itself." Differentiate this from volvulus, which is twisting itself.

Content Area: Child Health; **Category of Health Alteration:** Gastrointestinal Management; **Integrated Processes:** Nursing Process Analysis; **Client Need:** Physiological Integrity/Physiological Adaptation/Pathophysiology; **Cognitive Level:** Analysis; **Reference:** Pillitteri, A. (2010). pp. 1339–1344; **EBP Reference:** Sagar, J., Kumar, V., & Shah, D. (2006). Meckel's diverticulum: A systematic review. *Journal of the Royal Society of Medicine, 99*(10), 501–505.

227. During the afternoon shift report, an oncoming shift nurse is reviewing the documentation completed by a day shift nurse in the medical record of a 16-year-old client with ulcerative colitis (see exhibit). Which statement should the oncoming shift nurse most definitely clarify with the nurse from the previous shift?

NURSE'S NARRATIVE NOTES

1. 0830 Ate 75% of low protein and carbohydrate meal of bran muffin, milk, and orange juice._____ J. Dunn, RN

2. 0900 Antispasmotic agent given before breakfast is effective. Denies abdominal pain and cramping after eating. _____ J. Dunn, RN

3. 1300 Before administration, the client and parent were instructed on the purpose of azathioprine (Imuran), which is being used to wean the client off of steroids._____ J. Dunn, RN

4. 1430 Four loose bloody stools this shift. Client taught on use and application of barrier cream to protect the skin. _____ J. Dunn, RN

---

228. A nurse is collecting stool for a culture and sensitivity for ova and parasites to evaluate for the presence of bacterial gastroenteritis for a 6-month-old infant. Place each step in the correct numerical order (1–8) that the nurse should perform to correctly complete the procedure.

_____ 1. Document the specimen collection and action taken to deliver the specimen to the laboratory.

_____ 2. Use the sterile cotton swab to scrape a fresh, warm specimen of stool from the diaper.

_____ 3. Assemble exam gloves, identification label, sterile culture tube, sterile applicator (swab), and biohazard container.

_____ 4. Label the culture tube and the biohazard bag with the client's identification information, date, and specimen collected.

_____ 5. Don examination gloves.

_____ 6. Place the cotton swab in the sterile culture tube.

_____ 7. Deliver the stool specimen to the laboratory.

_____ 8. Remove gloves and perform hand hygiene.

227. ANSWER: 1.

A nurse should clarify an incorrect action. The diet used in the treatment of ulcerative colitis should be high in protein and carbohydrates with normal fat and decreased roughage. Antispasmodic agents should be administered before meals. Azathioprine, an immunomodulatory agent, is used to wean the client off of steroids. Ulcerative colitis is characterized by bloody diarrhea. The frequency of bloody stools can result in excoriation and skin breakdown. A barrier cream can help to protect the skin.

TEST-TAKING TIP: Consider the client's diagnosis. The key phrase is "most definitely clarify" which suggests that either an action is incorrect or the documentation is incorrect.

Content Area: Child Health; **Category of Health Alteration:** Gastrointestinal Management; **Integrated Processes:** Nursing Process Evaluation; **Client Need:** Physiological Integrity/Physiological Adaptation/Illness Management; **Cognitive Level:** Analysis; **Reference:** Ward, S., & Hisley, S. (2009), p. 795.

228. ANSWER: 3, 5, 2, 6, 8, 4, 7, 1.

First, assemble exam gloves, identification label, sterile culture tube, sterile applicator (swab), and biohazard container. Next, don examination gloves and then scrape a fresh, warm specimen of stool from the diaper using a sterile cotton swab. Place the cotton swab in the sterile culture tube and then remove gloves and perform hand hygiene. Label the culture tube and the biohazard bag with the client's identification information, date, and specimen collected. Next, deliver the stool specimen to the laboratory. Finally, document the specimen collection and action taken to deliver the specimen to the laboratory.

TEST-TAKING TIP: Identify the beginning and ending steps first and number these as 1 and 8. Of the remaining steps, visualize the procedure to place the actions in the correct sequence.

Content Area: Child Health; **Category of Health Alteration:** Gastrointestinal Management; **Integrated Processes:** Nursing Process Implementation; **Client Need:** Physiological Integrity/Reduction of Risk Potential/Diagnostic Tests; **Cognitive Level:** Application; **Reference:** Ward, S., & Hisley, S. (2009), p. 801.

Test 32: Child Health: Hematological and Oncological Management

229. A nurse is completing discharge teaching with the parents of a hospitalized 4-year-old child newly diagnosed with sickle cell disease. Which statements made by the parents indicate that teaching has been effective? **Select all that apply.**

1. "We plan to make arrangements to have genetic testing because we had planned to have more children."
2. "My child will need to be scheduled for pneumococcal, influenza, and meningococcal vaccinations."
3. "If my child develops a cold I should call the health care provider (HCP) immediately for antibiotic treatment."
4. "My child will need to be brought to the clinic for monthly blood transfusions after discharge."
5. "I should call the HCP if my child has dyspnea or other signs of acute chest syndrome."

230. A nurse is reviewing the serum laboratory report for a 2-year-old child with aplastic anemia secondary to chemotherapy treatments. Which findings should lead the nurse to conclude that treatment for aplastic anemia is effective? Place an X in the appropriate column to indicate that treatment is effective.

SERUM LABORATORY TEST RESULTS

Test	Client Results	Results Indicative of Resolving Pancytopenia
Hgb	10.5 g/dL	
RBC	4.9 m/mm³	
Plt	260,000/mm³	
WBC	5,900/mm³	
SCr	1.1 mg/dL	
BUN	31 mg/dL	
Glucose	107 mg/dL	

229. ANSWER: 1, 2, 3, 5.

Genetic testing is important because when both parents carry the trait, there is a 25% chance with each pregnancy of having a child with the disease. Because infection increases the risk of a sickle cell crisis, vaccinations are administered. Prophylaxis with antibiotics significantly reduces the risk of pneumococcal and other infections. Acute chest syndrome occurs from pulmonary infiltrate of abnormal blood cells and can lead to pulmonary failure and death. Early in the disease, every-3-week blood transfusions may be unnecessary. If the child experiences a stroke, transfusions would be given every 3 weeks on an ongoing basis.

TEST-TAKING TIP: Read each option carefully. Note that the child is newly diagnosed. Eliminate option 4 because it would not pertain to a child newly diagnosed with the disease.

Content Area: Child Health; **Category of Health Alteration:** Hematological and Oncological Management; **Integrated Processes:** Teaching and Learning; **Client Need:** Physiological Integrity/Physiological Adaptation/Illness Management; **Cognitive Level:** Analysis; **Reference:** Perry, S., Hockenberry, M., Lowdermilk, D., & Wilson, D. (2010), pp. 1495–1500.

230. ANSWER:

Test	Client Results	Results Indicative of Resolving Pancytopenia
Hgb	10.5 g/dL	X
RBC	4.9 m/mm³	X
Plt	260,000/mm³	X
WBC	5,900/mm³	X

Pancytopenia is a reduction in all cellular elements of the blood. Treatment is effective when the hemoglobin (Hgb), red blood cells (RBCs), platelets (Plt), and white blood cells (WBCs) return to a normal range for a 2-year-old child. Serum creatinine (SCr), blood urea nitrogen (BUN), and serum glucose are normal, but these values are not blood cell components.

TEST-TAKING TIP: Select only the laboratory values that reflect cellular elements of the blood and eliminate the other laboratory value choices.

Content Area: Child Health; **Category of Health Alteration:** Hematological and Oncological Management; **Integrated Processes:** Nursing Process Evaluation; **Client Need:** Physiological Integrity/Reduction of Risk Potential/Laboratory Values; **Cognitive Level:** Analysis; **Reference:** Ward, S., & Hisley, S. (2009), pp. 1074, 1087–1088.

231. A child is hospitalized with a severe viral infection. Which assessment findings should lead a nurse to conclude that the client is experiencing a potential complication of disseminated intravascular coagulation (DIC)? **Select all that apply.**

1. Hematemesis
2. Epistaxis
3. Purpura
4. Hypertension
5. Petechia

232. An experienced nurse orienting a new nurse is explaining the phases of chemotherapy treatments for an 8-year-old child just starting treatment for acute lymphocytic leukemia (ALL). In which order should the experienced nurse explain the phases of chemotherapy treatment? Place each step in the correct numerical order (1–4) in which the nurse should explain the four phases for chemotherapy administration.

_____ 1. Consolidation phase administering L-asparaginase and daunorubicin

_____ 2. Induction phase administering prednisone, vincristine, L-asparaginase, and daunorubicin

_____ 3. Maintenance of remission phase administering 6-mercaptopurine, 6-thioguanine, and methotrexate

_____ 4. Delayed intensification phase administering vincristine, cytosine arabinoside, and cyclophosphamide

231. ANSWER: 1, 2, 3, 5.

The presence of an underlying primary illness can place a child at high risk for developing DIC. Abnormal coagulation in DIC can lead to excessive bleeding, such as vomiting blood (hematemesis) and nose bleeds (epistaxis). Other signs of bleeding include purpura (appearance of red or purple discolorations on the skin from bleeding) and petechiae (pinpoint, flat round red spots under the skin surface caused by intradermal hemorrhage). Hypotension (not hypertension) may occur due to bleeding.

TEST-TAKING TIP: Consider that all options except one are associated with active blood loss, thus eliminate option 4.

Content Area: Child Health; **Category of Health Alteration:** Hematological and Oncological Management; **Integrated Processes:** Nursing Process Analysis; **Client Need:** Physiological Integrity/Reduction of Risk Potential/Potential for Complications from Surgical Procedures and Health Alterations; **Cognitive Level:** Application; **Reference:** Ward, S., & Hisley, S. (2009). pp. 1086–1087.

232. ANSWER: 2, 1, 4, 3.

Chemotherapy for ALL is divided into four phases. The first phase is the induction phase administering prednisone, vincristine, L-asparaginase, and daunorubicin. The second phase is the consolidation phase administering L-asparaginase, and daunorubicin. The third phase is the delayed intensification phase administering vincristine, cytosine arabinoside, and cyclophosphamide. The final phase is the maintenance of remission phase administering 6-mercaptopurine, 6-thioguanine, and methotrexate.

TEST-TAKING TIP: Use key words in the phases listed to put them in the appropriate sequence, e.g., "induction" and "maintenance." Knowing the chemotherapeutic agents in each phase is irrelevant to placing the phases in the correct order. However, exposure to the names of chemotherapeutic agents will assist you in recognizing them should they appear on the NCLEX-RN® examination.

Content Area: Child Health; **Category of Health Alteration:** Hematological and Oncological Management; **Integrated Processes:** Teaching and Learning; **Client Need:** Physiological Integrity/Physiological Adaptation/Illness Management; **Cognitive Level:** Application; **Reference:** Ball, J., & Bindler, R. (2008). p. 888; **EBP Reference:** Jost, L., Stahel, R., ESMO Guidelines Task Force. (2005). ESMO Minimum Clinical Recommendations for diagnosis, treatment and follow-up of Hodgkin's disease. *Annals of Oncology* (Suppl 1), 54–55.

233. A pediatric client weighing 66 pounds is to receive filgrastim (Neupogen) 5 mcg/kg subcutaneously for treatment of neutropenia. The medication vial contains 300 mcg per 1 mL. In order to give the correct dose, how many milliliters (mL) should the nurse prepare to administer?

_____ mL (Record your answer to the nearest tenth.)

234. A hospice nurse notifies family members of a 7-year-old child that the child's death is imminent. Which assessment findings prompted the nurse to conclude that the child's death is near? **Select all that apply.**

1. Cheyne-Stokes respirations
2. States seeing an angel coming to take him or her away
3. States that he or she is dying
4. A decrease in the volume of Korotkoff's sounds
5. Extremities feel warm to touch
6. Body is held in a rigid, unchanging position

233. ANSWER: 0.5
Use the proportion method to calculate the correct dosage:

<u>First, convert pounds to kilograms.</u>

2.2 pounds : 1 kg :: 66 pounds : X kg (multiply the outside values and then the inside values and solve for X).

2.2 X = 66 X = 30 kg

<u>Next, determine the dose:</u> **5 mcg $\times$ 30 kg = 150 mcg**

<u>Finally, determine the amount:</u> **300 mcg : 1 mL :: 150 mcg : X mL**

300 X = 150 X = 0.5 mL

TEST-TAKING TIP: Focus on the information in the question and use the on-screen calculator to calculate the correct dosage.

Content Area: Child Health; **Category of Health Alteration:** Hematological and Oncological Management; **Integrated Processes:** Nursing Process Implementation; **Client Need:** Physiological Integrity/Pharmacological and Parenteral Therapies/ Dosage Calculation; **Cognitive Level:** Analysis; **References:** Pickar, G., & Abernethy, A. (2008), p. 46; Wilson, B., Shannon, M., & Shields, K. (2010), pp. 648–650.

234. ANSWER: 1, 2, 3, 4, 6.
Physical and psychological signs that death is imminent include Cheyne-Stokes respirations, reports of seeing persons or objects not visible to others, stating he or she is dying, and a rigid body position. A decrease in the volume of Korotkoff's sounds during blood pressure auscultation and a change in pulse pressure indicate imminent death. Additional physical signs affect multiple body systems, including musculoskeletal, GI, respiratory, cardiovascular, neurological, and renal systems. Extremities will feel cold to touch, not warm, and show mottling with imminent death.

TEST-TAKING TIP: Recall that besides physical signs of imminent death, the client may express feelings of impending death.

Content Area: Child Health; **Category of Health Alteration:** Hematological and Oncological Management; **Integrated Processes:** Nursing Process Evaluation; **Client Need:** Psychosocial Integrity/End of Life Care; **Cognitive Level:** Application; **Reference:** Ball, J., & Bindler, R. (2008), p. 459; **EBP Reference:** Institute for Clinical Systems Improvement. (2008). *Palliative Care.* Retrieved from www.guideline.gov/ summary/summary.aspx?doc_id=12618&nbr=6526.

235. A nurse reads in a pediatric client's chart that the client has tinea corporis. When assessing the client, which skin condition should the nurse expect to observe?

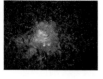

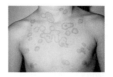

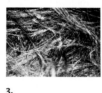

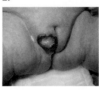

1.

2.

3.

4.

236. A nurse is assessing a 6-year-old child who had an acute onset of malaise, fever, and irritability followed by the rash illustrated and pruritus. Which question is **best** for the nurse to ask the parent?

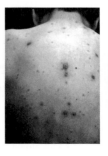

1. "Did your child receive immunizations for measles, mumps, and rubella (MMR)?"
2. "Have you been using baking soda or oatmeal baths to manage your child's itching?"
3. "Was your child exposed to someone with chickenpox in the last 7 days?"
4. "Did the lesions first appear on your child's extremities and then spread to the trunk?"

235. ANSWER: 2.
Tinea (ringworm) is a fungal skin disease occurring on various parts of the body. Option 2 shows tinea corporis occurring on the child's trunk.
Option 1 is tinea capitis, a fungal infection of the scalp. Option 3 is pediculosis capitis, a lice infestation of the hair and scalp. Option 4 is a hemangioma, a vascular tumor.

TEST-TAKING TIP: Tinea is ringworm. Use this clue to narrow the options to options 1 and 2.

Content Area: Child Health; **Category of Health Alteration:** Integumentary Management and Other Health Alterations; **Integrated Processes:** Nursing Process Assessment; **Client Need:** Physiological Integrity/Physiological Adaptation/Alterations in Body Systems; **Cognitive Level:** Application; **Reference:** Ball, J., & Bindler, R. (2008), pp. 1277–1282.

236. ANSWER: 2.
The rash illustrated is chickenpox caused by a varicella-zoster virus. It begins with a macule on a red base and progresses to clear vesicles that later form a crust. Pruritus is itching. Baking soda, oatmeal baths, and calamine lotion can be used to manage itching. The varicella and not the MMR vaccine is given to prevent chickenpox. Although asking about the MMR vaccine may help determine whether the child has had any immunizations, it is not the best option. The incubation period is from 13 to 17 days (not 7 days). The lesions generally first appear on the face and trunk (not the extremities) but may spread anywhere on the body.

TEST-TAKING TIP: Note that the appearance of the rash is a macule on a red base. Use this information to narrow the options. The key word is "best."

Content Area: Child Health; **Category of Health Alteration:** Integumentary Management and Other Health Alterations; **Integrated Processes:** Nursing Process Assessment; **Client Need:** Physiological Integrity/Physiological Adaptation/Alterations in Body Systems; **Cognitive Level:** Analysis; **Reference:** Ward, S., & Hisley, S. (2009), pp. 82, 832.

237. A nurse completed teaching for the parents and their 6-year-old child who has just been diagnosed with impetigo. Which statements by a parent indicate that teaching was effective? **Select all that apply.**

1. "Because impetigo is a highly contagious bacterial infection, I should keep my child home from school for 24 hours after the start of the oral antibiotic."
2. "I should ensure that my child completes the full 3-day course of the dicloxacillin (Dynapen) antibiotic."
3. "Because this is a viral infection, topical antibiotics will be ineffective, but the lesions will dry and scab over in a few days."
4. "I will need to be sure to stress the importance of hand washing and not scratching the lesions because the lesions are very contagious."
5. "Although the impetigo is on my child's face, I should check my child's hands, neck, trunk, buttocks, and extremities because these are other areas where it can also appear."

238. A child has a partial-thickness scald burn to the chest and both arms. Which interventions should the nurse expect when planning care for the child? **Select all that apply.**

1. Prepare the child for a whirlpool bath.
2. Administer morphine sulfate 0.1 mg/kg IV 15 minutes prior to a dressing change.
3. Scrub the burned area to remove dead tissue and topical medications.
4. Reinforce dressings that have become saturated with exudate.
5. Apply antibacterial agents such as topical silver sulfadiazine (Silvadene) to the burned area.

237. ANSWER: 1, 4, 5.

Impetigo is a highly contagious bacterial infection. Oral antibiotics are used if the infection is widespread and the child is required to stay home from school for 24 hours after initiating the oral antibiotic. Careful hand hygiene and avoiding scratching of the lesions will help to prevent the spread of the infection. Although the lesions are most commonly found on and around the mouth or elsewhere on the face, impetigo can also appear on the hands, neck, trunk, buttocks, or extremities. A full course of dicloxacillin is 7 days, not 3 days. Impetigo is a bacterial, not a viral, infection.

TEST-TAKING TIP: Examine options 1 and 3 first, because these address different causative organisms. Eliminate one of these options. Carefully read option 2 and eliminate this option after considering that a full-course of antibiotics would be longer than 3 days.

Content Area: Child Health; **Category of Health Alteration:** Integumentary Management and Other Health Alterations; **Integrated Processes:** Teaching and Learning; **Client Need:** Health Promotion and Maintenance/Principles of Teaching and Learning; **Cognitive Level:** Application; **Reference:** Ward, S., & Hisley, S. (2009), p. 1006.

238. ANSWER: 1, 2, 5.

Whirlpool baths (hydrotherapy) are given to cleanse extensive wounds before débridement, to increase vasodilation and circulation, and to enhance healing. Dressing changes are often painful, so pharmacological pain management is needed. The dose is appropriate. Antibacterial agents are applied to partial-thickness burns. Newer silver-based antimicrobial dressings provide sustained release delivery of silver. Gently washing (not scrubbing) is necessary to protect new epithelial cells. Dressings should be changed if they become soiled with exudate.

TEST-TAKING TIP: Eliminate any options that increase the child's risk of injury or infection.

Content Area: Child Health; **Category of Health Alteration:** Integumentary Management and Other Health Alterations; **Integrated Processes:** Nursing Process Planning; **Client Need:** Physiological Integrity/Reduction of Risk Potential/Therapeutic Procedures; **Cognitive Level:** Application; **Reference:** Ball, J., & Bindler, R. (2008), pp. 480, 1289.

239. A nurse is reviewing laboratory results for a 10-year-old child who is admitted with a diagnosis of chickenpox. Which value should be **most** concerning to the nurse?

Serum Laboratory Test	Client's Value	Normal Levels
Blood urea nitrogen	25 mg/dL	5–25 mg/dL
Creatinine	1.6 mg/dL	0.5–1.5 mg/ dL
Sodium	133 mg/dL	135–145 mEq/L
Potassium	3.4 mg/dL	3.5–5.3 mEq/L
Chloride	110 mg/dL	95–105 mEq/L
Platelets	90,000/mm³	150,000–450,000/mm³

1. Platelets, because it can increase the risk for bleeding.
2. Potassium, because low potassium can impact cardiac function.
3. Sodium, because it increases the risk for seizures.
4. Creatinine, because it is indicative of decreased renal function.

240. A nurse is preparing to administer amphotericin B deoxycholate (Fungizone) 1 mg/kg intravenously (IV) now for the treatment of a severe fungal infection. The child weighs 55 pounds. The medication is prepared in a 50-mg vial of powder that must be reconstituted with 10 mL of sterile water before being diluted in 250 mL of D5W for IV administration over 30 to 60 minutes. How many milliliters (mL) of the medication should the nurse add to the 250 mL bag of D5W to administer the correct dose of medication?

_____ mL (Record your answer as a whole number.)

239. ANSWER: 1.

Thrombocytopenia (low platelet count) is a common complication of chickenpox. Low platelets can increase the risk for bleeding. Ten percent of children with chickenpox will develop a complication. There are other laboratory tests that are concerning but not as important as the platelet count. Potassium is low and serum creatinine is elevated, but these levels are not the most concerning because they are near normal. Low serum sodium levels can produce seizures, but this value is borderline low.

TEST-TAKING TIP: Review the chart carefully and think of the laboratory value alterations that could be indicative of complications from chicken pox.

Content Area: Child Health; **Category of Health Alteration:** Integumentary Management and Other Health Alterations; **Integrated Processes:** Nursing Process Analysis; **Client Need:** Physiological Integrity Reduction of Risk Potential/Laboratory Values; **Cognitive Level:** Analysis; **References:** Pillitteri, A. (2010), pp. 1268–1269; Ward, S., & Hisley, S. (2009), p. 832.

240. ANSWER: 5.

Use a proportion formula, multiply the inside and then the outside values, and solve for *X*:

First, convert pounds to kilograms:

1 kg : 2.2 pounds : *X* kg : 55 lbs; 2.2 *X* = 55; *X* = 25 (55 lbs = 25 kg)

Next, determine the dose in mg:

1 kg : 1 mg :: 25 kg: *X* mg; *X* = 25 mg

Finally, determine the milliliters of reconstituted medication that should be added to the 250 mL of D5W:

50 mg : 10 mL :: 25 mg : *X* mL; 50 *X* = 250; *X* = 5 mL

5 mL of reconstituted medication should be added to the 250 mL of D5W to administer the correct dose.

TEST-TAKING TIP: With a complex question such as this, first determine what the question is asking. Next convert pounds to kilograms, determine the dose in milligrams, and then determine the amount in milliliters.

Content Area: Child Health; **Category of Health Alteration:** Integumentary Management and Other Health Alterations; **Integrated Processes:** Nursing Process Implementation; **Client Need:** Physiological Integrity/Pharmacological and Parenteral Therapies/Dosage Calculation; **Cognitive Level:** Analysis; **References:** Deglin, J., & Vallerand, A. (2011), pp. 165–169; Ward, S., & Hisley, S. (2009), p. 844.

241. A nurse is palpating the fontanels of an infant hospitalized with a head injury. Which area should the nurse palpate to assess the posterior fontanel? Place an X on the posterior fontanel.

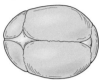

242. A nurse is completing a health history and physical assessment for a 4-year-old child who has spastic-type cerebral palsy (CP). Which statements made by a parent during the assessment should prompt the nurse to conclude that the parents have a good understanding of their child's condition? **Select all that apply.**

1. "I perform range of motion (ROM) exercises every 4 hours to help prevent contractures."
2. "I give my child a therapeutic massage after the stretching exercises to help manage the pain."
3. "I minimize the calories I provide with meals because my child is more prone to obesity."
4. "I have my child wear a helmet during the day because of chronic tonic-clonic seizures."
5. "Using utensils with large, padded handles makes it easier for my child to feed himself."

241. ANSWER:

The posterior fontanel is the smaller of the two fontanels. Fullness of the fontanels is a potential sign of increased intracranial pressure.

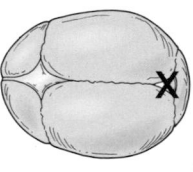

TEST-TAKING TIP: Focus on the size of the fontanels.

Content Area: Child Health; **Category of Health Alteration:** Neurological and Musculoskeletal Management; **Integrated Processes:** Nursing Process Assessment; **Client Need:** Physiological Integrity/Physiological Adaptation/Alterations in Body Systems; **Cognitive Level:** Application; **Reference:** Ward, S., & Hisley, S. (2009), p. 674.

242. ANSWER: 1, 2, 4, 5.

A child with spastic CP has hypertonia and rigidity and is prone to contractures; ROM exercises every 4 hours are essential to maintain joint flexibility and to prevent contractures. Therapeutic massage can help to control the pain associated with spasticity and stretching exercises. A child with chronic tonic-clonic seizures should wear a helmet to protect against a head injury. Utensils with large, padded handles are appropriate for a child with spasticity and promote the child's independence in eating. A child with CP requires high-calorie diets and sometimes supplements because of feeding difficulties associated with spasticity.

TEST-TAKING TIP: Eliminate the one option that is different from the other options.

Content Area: Child Health; **Category of Health Alteration:** Neurological and Musculoskeletal Management; **Integrated Processes:** Nursing Process Evaluation; **Client Need:** Health Promotion and Maintenance/Self-care; **Cognitive Level:** Application; **Reference:** Ball, J., & Bindler, R. (2008), pp. 1076–1081.

243. A nurse performs a neurological assessment on a 1-year-old child using the Glasgow coma scale. The child does not open his or her eyes when the nurse walks into the room and then calls the child's name. When pressure is applied to the child's orbital notch, the child opens his or her eyes and tries to withdraw from the pain stimulus. With stimulation, the child becomes more restless, but does not cry. Which score should the nurse document in the child's medical record?

_____. (Record your answer as a whole number.)

NEUROLOGICAL ASSESSMEMT

Pupils	Right	Size		++ = Brisk
		Reaction		+ = Sluggish
	Left	Size		— = No reaction
		Reaction		C = Eye closed by swelling

Eyes open	Spontaneously	4	
	To speech	3	
	To pain	2	
	None	1	

Best motor response	Obeys commands	6	Usually record best arm or age-appropriate response
	Localizes pain	5	
	Flexion withdrawal	4	
	Flexion abnormal	3	
	Extension	2	
	None	1	

Pupil scale (mm)

• 1
• 2
● 3
● 4
● 5
● 6
● 7
● 8

Best response to auditory and/or visual stimulus	>2 years		<2 years
	Orientation	5	5 Smiles, listens, follows
	Confused	4	4 Cries, consolable
	Inappropriate words	3	3 Inappropriate persistent cry
	Incomprehensible words	2	2 Agitated, restless
	None	1	1 No response
	Endotracheal tube or trach	T	

COMA SCALE TOTAL	

GLASGOW SCALE TOTAL

243. ANSWER: 8.

When pressure is applied to the child's orbital notch, the child opens his or her eyes (2), tries to withdraw from the pain stimulus (4), and with stimulation, the child becomes more restless (2).

TEST-TAKING TIP: Carefully read the scenario and then compare the child's reaction to the Glasgow coma scale. Be sure to use the scale for <2 years.

Content Area: Child Health; **Category of Health Alteration:** Neurological and Musculoskeletal Management; **Integrated Processes:** Communication and Documentation; **Client Need:** Physiological Integrity/Reduction of Risk Potential/ System Specific Assessment; **Cognitive Level:** Application; **Reference:** Ward, S., & Hisley, S. (2009), p. 923.

244. A child has a newly applied fiberglass hip-spica cast. Which interventions should the nurse include when caring for the child? **Select all that apply.**

1. Use a hair dryer to promote drying of the child's cast.
2. Place the child on a Bradford Frame to elevate the child off the bed.
3. Place pillows to support the child's lower extremities.
4. Turn the child every 2 hours.
5. Petal the perineal area of the hip-spica cast.
6. Assess the circulation, motion, and sensation (CMS) of the child's feet hourly.

245. A nurse is planning care for an infant born with spina bifida. Which important management concerns should the nurse include in the plan of care? **Select all that apply.**

1. Careful management of protruding segments of the bowel
2. Careful management of a protruding bladder
3. Careful management of protruding spinal cord contents
4. Careful management to prevent contamination of the defect site by bowel and bladder contents
5. Careful management of talipes equinovarus

244. ANSWER: 3, 4, 5.
A fiberglass cast dries within 30 minutes. Pillows are used to support the lower extremities to prevent pressure areas. Turning every 2 hours prevents cast syndrome. Petaling (applying waterproof adhesive tape to the edges of the cast) protects the cast from soiling. Hair dryers should never be used to promote drying because the heat can result in burn injuries. A child with a plaster of Paris hip-spica cast is placed on a Bradford Frame, which elevates the child off the bed and facilitates drying. Plaster of Paris casts take 10 to 72 hours to dry. Although CMS should be assessed after cast application, this is an assessment and not an intervention.

TEST-TAKING TIP: Recall that fiberglass casts dry quicker than plaster of Paris casts. Eliminate options that would cause injury, the one that pertains to a plaster of Paris cast, and the one that is an assessment and not an intervention.

Content area: Child Health; **Category of Health Alteration:** Neurological and Musculoskeletal Management; **Integrated Processes:** Nursing Process Implementation; **Client Need:** Physiological Integrity/Basic Care and Comfort/Mobility/Immobility; **Cognitive Level:** Application; **Reference:** Ward, S., & Hisley, S. (2009), pp. 965–966.

245. ANSWER: 3, 4.
The careful management of protruding spinal cord contents and the prevention of the defect site from contamination by bowel and bladder contents are important nursing concerns when caring for an infant born with spina bifida. Segments of the bowel or bladder do not protrude in spina bifida. Talipes equinovarus is a clubfoot and not associated with spina bifida.

TEST-TAKING TIP: Use the word "spina" and a clue to selecting the correct options.

Content area: Child Health; **Category of Health Alteration:** Neurological and Musculoskeletal Management; **Integrated Processes:** Nursing Process Analysis; **Client Need:** Physiological Integrity/Physiological Adaptation/Illness Management; **Cognitive Level:** Application; **Reference:** Ball, J., & Bindler, R. (2008), pp. 1066–1069.

Test 35: Child Health: Renal and Urinary Management

246. A nurse is evaluating whether treatment is effective for an 8-year-old client with chronic renal failure who is receiving sevelamer hydrochloride (Renagel). Place an X on the laboratory test results that indicate that the treatment is effective.

Serum Laboratory Test	Client's Value	Normal Values
Potassium	4.0 mEq/L	3.4–4.7 mEq/L
Calcium	9.2 mg/dL	8.8–10.8 mg/dL
Phosphorus	5.0 g/dL	3.7–5.6 mg/dL
Albumin	4.0 g/dL	3.7–5.1 g/dL
Red blood cells (RBCs)	4.9 m/mm^3	3.89–4.96 m/mm^3
Hemoglobin (Hgb)	12 g/dL	10.2–13.4 g/dL
Hematocrit (Hct)	40%	31.7%–39.3%

247. A nurse completed teaching for a sexually active, female adolescent with recurrent urinary tract infections (UTIs) on strategies to prevent reoccurrence. Which statements made by the adolescent indicates that the nurse's teaching was effective? **Select all that apply**.

1. "I should void after intercourse."
2. "I should drink 64 ounces of water daily."
3. "I should be wearing silk underwear."
4. "I should be taking showers instead of baths."
5. "I should apply powder to the perineal area before intercourse."
6. "I should be sure that my partner uses a latex condom."

246. ANSWER:

Calcium	9.2 mg/dL **X**	8.8–10.8 mg/dL
Phosphorus	5.0 g/dL **X**	3.7–5.6 mg/dL

Sevelamer hydrochloride reduces absorption of phosphorus from the intestines. It will elevate the serum calcium level, thus decreasing the serum phosphorus level. Phosphorus is elevated in chronic renal failure because the kidneys are unable to excrete it.

TEST-TAKING TIP: If unsure, consider the kidney's role in excreting phosphorus and the inverse relationship between phosphorus and calcium.

Content Area: Child Health; **Category of Health Alteration:** Renal & Urinary Management; **Integrated Processes:** Nursing Process Evaluation; **Client Need:** Physiological Integrity/Pharmacological and Parenteral Therapies/Expected Actions or Outcomes; **Cognitive Level:** Analysis; **References:** Ball, J., & Bindler, R. (2008), pp. 1000–1001, 1322–1323; Ward, S., & Hisley, S. (2009), p. 1055.

247. ANSWER: 1, 2, 4.

Voiding after intercourse, drinking 64 ounces of water daily, and taking showers rather than baths are strategies to prevent recurrent UTIs. Applying powder to the perineal area is not recommended, as it may increase the likelihood of infection. Cotton underwear is recommended, rather than silk. While condoms may prevent STDs, they do not prevent UTIs.

TEST-TAKING TIP: Select options that should be nonirritating and prevent bacterial growth.

Content Area: Child Health; **Category of Health Alteration:** Renal and Urinary Management; **Integrated Processes:** Nursing Process Evaluation; **Client Need:** Health Promotion and Maintenance/Disease Prevention; **Cognitive Level:** Application; **Reference:** Berman, A., Snyder, S., Kozier, B., & Erb, G. (2008), pp. 1298–1299.

248. A nurse is planning care for a child to be admitted for a hypospadias repair. Which illustration best reflects the nurse's critical thinking about the child's condition?

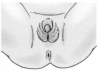

1.

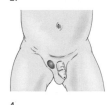

2.

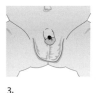

3.

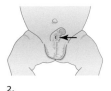

4.

249. A 6-year-old child is seen in a clinic with suspected cystitis. Which findings on a nurse's assessment are consistent with cystitis? **Select all that apply**.

1. Enuresis
2. Strong-smelling urine
3. Costovertebral angle tenderness
4. Hematuria
5. Suprapubic pain

248. ANSWER: 2.

Hypospadias is a congenital anomaly involving the abnormal location of the urethral meatus on the ventral surface of the penis. Option 1 is ambiguous genitalia in which external reproductive organs cannot be easily identified as male or female. Note the urethra on the testicle. In epispadias (option 3) the urethral canal is open on the dorsal surface of the penis. Option 4 is an undecended testicle and is unrelated to hypospadias.

TEST-TAKING TIP: Use the prefix "hypo-" as a cue to select the correct option.

Content Area: Child Health; **Category of Health Alteration:** Renal & Urinary Management; **Integrated Processes:** Nursing Process Planning; **Client Need:** Physiological Integrity/Physiological Adaptation/Pathophysiology; **Cognitive Level:** Application; **Reference:** Ball, J., & Bindler, R. (2008), pp. 983–985.

249. ANSWER: 1, 2, 4, 5.

Clinical manifestations of cystitis, a lower urinary tract infection (UTI), includes enuresis (bedwetting in a previously potty-trained child), strong-smelling urine from the accumulation of nitrates, and hematuria and suprapubic pain from the effects of the bacteria on the urethra and bladder wall. Costovertebral angle tenderness is seen with an upper UTI such as pyelonephritis.

TEST-TAKING TIP: Eliminate any option that pertains to an upper UTI.

Content Area: Child Health; **Category of Health Alteration:** Renal & Urinary Management; **Integrated Processes:** Nursing Process Assessment; **Client Need:** Physiological Integrity/Physiological Adaptation/Alterations in Body Systems; **Cognitive Level:** Application; **Reference:** Ball, J., & Bindler, R. (2008), p. 979.

250. An 18-month-old child with a history of fever, harsh cough, and excessive drooling is brought to an emergency department. A parent states the child has been teething and had a fever of 102.4°F (39.1°C) upon awakening this morning. The toddler's cry is raspier than a normal cry. A lateral neck radiograph shows evidence of epiglottitis. In the graphic below, place an X over the area where a nurse should expect to visualize the swollen epiglottis.

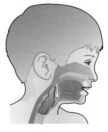

251. A nurse is assessing a 7-month-old infant diagnosed with pneumonia. Which signs and symptoms should the nurse conclude are related to the diagnosis? **Select all that apply.**

1. Productive cough with white sputum
2. Tachypnea
3. Rhonchi
4. Dullness on percussion
5. Excessive crying
6. Subnormal temperature

250. ANSWER:
The epiglottis is a flap of elastic cartilage tissue covered with a mucous membrane, attached to the root of the tongue. It projects obliquely upward behind the tongue and the hyoid bone. Understanding normal anatomy facilitates a nurse in defining diagnostic results and improves the nurse's ability to provide safe and effective treatment for the client.

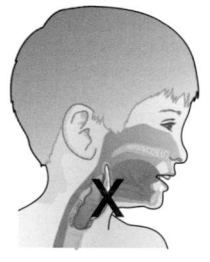

TEST-TAKING TIP: Examine your own or another's oral cavity for the size, position, and structure of the epiglottis to determine an average size and then look for a similar structure on the illustration.

Content Area: Child Health; **Category of Health Alteration:** Respiratory Management; **Integrated Processes:** Nursing Process Analysis; **Client Need:** Physiological Integrity/Physiological Adaptation/Pathophysiology; **Cognitive Level:** Application; **Reference:** Pillitteri, A. (2010), pp. 1165–1168.

251. ANSWER: 1, 2, 3, 4.
Coughing is due to the excessive sputum production with pneumonia. The blocked airways increase respiratory effort (tachypnea) and mucus in the airways causes scattered rhonchi throughout the lung fields. Consolidation causes dullness on percussion. Excessive crying is not usually noted; children are lethargic and listless. Children with pneumonia usually have high fever (not subnormal temperature) and are warm to the touch.

TEST-TAKING TIP: Focus on the condition and eliminate options opposite of what would be expected.

Content Area: Child Health; **Category of Health Alteration:** Respiratory Management; **Integrated Processes:** Nursing Process Assessment; **Client Need:** Physiological Integrity/Reduction of Risk Potential/System Specific Assessments; **Cognitive Level:** Application; **Reference:** Ball, J., & Bindler, R. (2008), pp. 705–706.

252. A nurse performs an injection on a 10-month-old hospitalized infant and leaves the needle cap within reach of the infant. The infant begins choking after placing the object in his or her mouth. Place each step in the correct numerical order (1–5) that the nurse should take to correctly perform the Heimlich maneuver.

_____ 1. Give five chest thrusts using two fingers at a distance of one fingerbreadth below the nipple line.

_____ 2. Give five blows to the infant's back using the heel of the hand.

_____ 3. Lay the infant on the nurse's thigh with the infant's head facing down.

_____ 4. Check the infant's mouth for any obvious presence of the object that can be removed.

_____ 5. Turn the infant over, face up.

253. A nurse is answering questions being asked by the parents of a 5-year-old child newly diagnosed with moderate persistent asthma. Which statements is the nurse likely to make in response to the parents' questions? **Select all that apply.**

1. "Skin testing can be performed to identify any allergens that can trigger an asthma attack."
2. "During an acute asthma episode, your child's respirations will be rapid and labored."
3. "Daily medications are not required, but your child would receive systemic corticosteroids when an asthma attack occurs."
4. "Your child is too young to use a peak expiratory flowmeter for identifying when an obstruction is occurring."
5. "Encasing your child's pillows and mattress in plastic covers can help to control dust mites in your child's bedroom."

252. ANSWER: 3, 2, 5, 1, 4.

First, lay the infant on the nurse's thigh with the infant's head facing down. Next, give five blows to the infant's back using the heel of the hand. Third, turn the infant over, face up. Fourth, give five chest thrusts using two fingers at a distance of one fingerbreadth below the nipple line. Finally, check the infant's mouth for any obvious presence of the object that can be removed.

TEST-TAKING TIP: Visualize the sequence of actions prior to placing these in the correct order.

Content Area: Child Health; **Category of Health Alteration:** Respiratory Management; **Integrated Processes:** Nursing Process Implementation; **Client Need:** Physiological Integrity/Physiological Adaptation/Medical Emergencies; **Cognitive Level:** Application; **Reference:** Ward, S., & Hisley, S. (2009), p. 776.

253. ANSWER: 1, 2, 5.

Skin testing may be performed to identify allergens that serve as asthma triggers. Respirations are rapid and labored, and nasal flaring and intercostal retractions may be visible during an acute asthma episode. Dust mites have the potential to trigger an asthma attack, and exposure can be minimized by encasing the pillows and mattress in plastic covers. The preferred treatment is daily use of a low- to medium-dose inhaled corticosteroid and a long-acting beta-2 agonist. A 5-year-old child is able to cooperate and follow instructions for using a peak expiratory flowmeter; a parent's assistance may be needed for assisting the child and recording the values.

TEST-TAKING TIP: Consider the type of asthma and the age of the child to eliminate options.

Content Area: Child Health; **Category of Health Alteration:** Respiratory Management; **Integrated Processes:** Communication and Documentation; **Client Need:** Physiological Integrity/Physiological Adaptation/Illness Management; **Cognitive Level:** Analysis; **Reference:** Ball, J., & Bindler, R. (2008), pp. 712–723.

254. A nurse is preparing for the admission of a 6-year-old client with cystic fibrosis (CF) who is being hospitalized with a *Burkholderia cepacia* (*B. cepacia*) infection. Which interventions should the nurse include in the plan of care for the child? **Select all that apply.**

1. Place the child in a room with another child with CF.
2. Administer pancreatic enzymes such as pancrelipase (Pancrease).
3. Teach the parents about camps for their child sponsored by the Cystic Fibrosis Foundation.
4. Arrange for chest physiotherapy three times daily before meals.
5. Initiate airborne precautions.
6. Teach the parents about the positive effects of performing massage therapy on their child.

255. A nurse is reviewing the laboratory results for a 6-year-old client hospitalized with asthma complicated by an upper respiratory infection. In evaluating the laboratory results, the nurse considers possible causes. Based on these values, which cause should the nurse rule out?

Serum Laboratory Test	Client's Value	Normal Values
BUN	28	5–18 mg/dL
Creatinine	0.5	0.3–0.7 mg/dL

1. Dehydration
2. Hemorrhage
3. Renal impairment
4. Corticosteroid therapy

254. ANSWER: 2, 4, 6.

Pancreatic enzymes assist in digestion of nutrients decreasing fat and bulk. Chest physiotherapy is usually performed one to three times per day before meals to clear secretions. Coughing during chest physiotherapy can stimulate vomiting. Research with parent-administered massage therapy has found positive benefits that include improvement in the child's quality of life, decreased child and parent anxiety, and improved child mood, peak airflow, and breathing. Children with CF are not co-roomed to reduce the risk for transfer of the infectious organism. Children infected with *B. cepacia* are not permitted to attend events or camps sponsored by the Cystic Fibrosis Foundation due to the risk of infecting those with CF who are not yet infected with *B. cepacia*. Droplet precautions should be initiated (not airborne).

TEST-TAKING TIP: Eliminate options that would increase the risk of transmission of *B. cepacia*, which is spread by droplets.

Content Area: Child Health; **Category of Health Alteration:** Respiratory Management; **Integrated Processes:** Nursing Process Planning; **Client Need:** Physiological Integrity/Physiological Adaptation/Illness Management; **Cognitive Level:** Analysis; **Reference:** Ball, J., & Bindler, R. (2008), pp. 728–733; **EBP References:** Cincinnati Children's Hospital Medical Center. (2009). *Best evidence statement* (BESt). *Cystic Fibrosis-Effects of Massage Therapy on Quality of Life*. Cincinnati, OH: Cincinnati Children's Hospital Medical Center. Retrieved from www.guideline.gov/summary/summary.aspx?doc_id=14578&nbr=007252&string=pain.

255. ANSWER: 3.

The serum creatinine is normal; the client is unlikely experiencing renal impairment. A client with an elevated BUN may be dehydrated, hemorrhaging, or be receiving corticosteroid therapy.

TEST-TAKING TIP: The key phrase is "rule out." Select the option that would result in an elevated serum creatinine along with the elevated BUN and eliminate options that only elevate the BUN level.

Content Area: Child Health; **Category of Health Alteration:** Respiratory Management; **Integrated Processes:** Nursing Process Evaluation; **Client Need:** Physiological Integrity/Reduction of Risk Potential/Laboratory Values; **Cognitive Level:** Analysis; **Reference:** Perry, S., Hockenberry, M., Lowdermilk, D., & Wilson, D. (2010), pp. 1530, 1542.

Test 37: Child Health: Pharmacological and Parenteral Therapies

256. A nurse is evaluating the effectiveness of Humalog and Lantus insulin being administered by the parents to a 2-year-old child with type 1 diabetes mellitus (DM). Which findings on the serum laboratory report indicate that treatment is effective? Place an X in the effective treatment column for the client's laboratory results reflecting that treatment is effective.

LABORATORY REPORT

Serum Laboratory Test	Client Result	Effective Treatment
Creatinine	0.9 mg/dL	
White blood cells (WBCs)	4,000/mm³	
Hemoglobin	11 g/dL	
Hemoglobin A$_{1C}$	4.5%	
Potassium	3.9 mEq/L	
Glucose	70 mg/dL	

257. A severely dehydrated school-age child is to receive 2,000 mL of intravenous fluid over the next 8 hours. At what rate in milliliters per hour (mL/hr) should the nurse set the infusion pump?

_____ mL/hr (Record your answer as a whole number.)

256. ANSWER:

LABORATORY REPORT

Serum Laboratory Test	Client Result	Effective Treatment
Hemoglobin A_{1C}	4.5%	X
Glucose	70 mg/dL	X

The goal of treatment for children with type 1 DM is that the blood glucose levels are maintained at a relatively normal level. Hemoglobin A_{1C} levels are indicative of the average blood glucose levels over the past 2 to 3 months. Although the other laboratory values are normal, these do not indicate the effectiveness of treatment with insulin.

TEST-TAKING TIP: Be sure to place the X on two of the laboratory results, one showing immediate treatment effectiveness and the other showing effective treatment over the previous 2 to 3 months.

Content Area: Child Health; **Category of Health Alteration:** Pharmacological and Parenteral Therapies; **Integrated Processes:** Nursing Process Evaluation; **Client Need:** Physiological Integrity/Pharmacological and Parenteral Therapies/ Expected Actions or Outcomes; **Cognitive Level:** Analysis; **Reference:** Ward, S., & Hisley, S. (2009). pp. 907–909.

257. ANSWER: 250
2,000 mL divided by 8 hours = 250 mL/hour.

TEST-TAKING TIP: Carefully read what the question is asking. This is a simple division problem.

Content Area: Child Health; **Category of Health Alteration:** Pharmacological and Parenteral Therapies; **Integrated Processes:** Nursing Process Implementation; **Client Need:** Physiological Integrity/Pharmacological and Parenteral Therapies/ Parenteral/Intravenous Therapies; **Cognitive Level:** Application; **Reference:** Pickar, G., & Abernethy, A. (2008). p. 374.

258. A new nurse is being observed administering medications to a pediatric client hospitalized with asthma and bronchial pneumonia. The child's oral temperature is 103°F (39.4°C). An experienced nurse determines that the new nurse appropriately applied principles of medical asepsis when administering the medications. Prioritize the order in which the new nurse should have administered the medications.

_____ 1. Acetaminophen (Tylenol) 10–15 mg/kg/dose rectal q4–6h prn

_____ 2. Cefuroxime sodium (Zinacef) 1.2 gm IVPB q8h

_____ 3. Nystatin (Mycostatin) 100,000 units PO suspension to affected areas of mouth tid

_____ 4. Methylprednisolone (Solu-Medrol) 25 mg IVP q6h

_____ 5. Albuterol sulfate (Proventil) 90 mcg per inhalation, 2 puffs q4h

_____ 6. Beclomethasone (Beclovent) 42 mcg/oral inhalation, 2 puffs q24h

258. ANSWER: 4, 2, 5, 6, 3, 1.

Using the principles of medical asepsis, the nurse should administer medications beginning with areas that are most clean. Because methyl-prednisolone is administered IV push over 1 to 2 minutes, it should be administered first. It is a systemic corticosteroid that decreases inflammation. Cefuroxime sodium is administered by IV piggyback over 30 minutes. It is a second-generation cephalosporin that binds to the penicillin-binding proteins located on the cell walls of susceptible microorganisms. Albuterol sulfate should be administered third. It is a beta-2 agonist bronchodilator most commonly used in rescue therapy for acute asthmatic symptoms. An inhaled bronchodilator should be administered before an inhaled steroid to ensure deeper penetration of the steroid into the airways. Beclomethasone is an inhaled corticosteroid that inhibits bronchoconstriction, relaxes smooth muscle, and may decrease the number and activity of inflammatory cells, thus decreasing airway hyperresponsiveness. A side effect of oral inhalation steroid use is thrush. Nystatin is an antifungal agent that changes the permeability of the fungal cell membrane causing cellular contents to leak and fungal cell death. It is applied topically to treat thrush that can occur from oral steroid use. Finally, a rectal medication should be administered last. Acetaminophen is an antipyretic.

TEST-TAKING TIP: When determining the order of medication administration, first apply the principles of asepsis and then consider how rapid medications can be administered and their effects. When medications are to be administered by the same route, the medications that take the least amount of time to administer should be given first.

Content Area: Child Health; **Category of Health Alteration:** Pharmacological and Parenteral Therapies; **Integrated Processes:** Nursing Process Evaluation; **Client Need:** Safe and Effective Care Environment/Safety and Infection Control/ Medical Surgical Asepsis; **Cognitive Level:** Analysis; **Reference:** Berman, A., Snyder, S., Kozier, B., & Erb, G. (2008). p. 681.

259. A 6-year-old child is admitted to an emergency department in an unresponsive state. A parent states that an empty prescription container of hydrocodone 5 mg/acetaminophen 500 mg (Lorcet) was lying next to the child's bed. Which medications should a nurse anticipate administering to the child? **Select all that apply.**

1. Flumazenil (Romazicon)
2. Sodium bicarbonate
3. Naloxone (Narcan)
4. Vitamin K
5. Acetylcysteine (N-Acetylcysteine)

260. A nurse is preparing to administer fosphenytoin (Cerebyx) 2 mg PE/kg intravenously (IV) to a 5-year-old child hospitalized with a seizure disorder. The medication is available in a 50 mg PE/mL vial. The child weighs 44 pounds. How many milliliters of medication should the nurse prepare to administer?

_____ mL (Record your answer to the nearest tenth.)

259. ANSWER: 3, 5.

Lorcet contains hydrocodone, an opiate analgesic, and acetaminophen. Naloxone, a narcotic antagonist, reverses the effects of opiates. The antidote for acetaminophen poisoning is N-Acetylcysteine (NAC). NAC prevents liver damage and has anti-inflammatory, antioxidant, and positive inotropic effects. Flumazenil antagonizes the effects of benzodiazepines on the central nervous system (CNS) which cause sedation, impaired recall, and psychomotor impairment. Sodium bicarbonate, an alkalinizing agent, is an antidote for tricyclic antidepressant or lithium carbonate overdose. Vitamin K is an antidote for warfarin overdose.

TEST-TAKING TIP: Lorcet is a combination medication. Select the antidotes for both an opiate and acetaminophen overdose.

Content Area: Child Health; **Category of Health Alteration:** Pharmacological and Parenteral Therapies; **Integrated Processes:** Nursing Process Planning; **Client Need:** Physiological Integrity/Pharmacological and Parenteral Therapies/Expected Effects/ Outcomes; **Cognitive Level:** Application; **Reference:** Wilson, B., Shannon, M., Shields, K., & Stang, C. (2008), pp. 15–16, 649–650, 1044–1045, 1392–1393, 1654.

260. ANSWER: 0.8

First, convert the pounds to kilograms. Use a proportion formula, and then multiply the outside values and the inside values.

2.2 pounds : 1 kg :: 44 pounds : X kg

$2.2X = 44$

$X = 20$.

Next, calculate the dose: $2 \times 20 = 40$ mg

Finally, calculate the amount: 50 mg : 1 mL :: 40 mg : X mL

$50X = 40$

$X = 0.8$ mL

TEST-TAKING TIP: Use the conversion 2.2 pounds equals 1 kilogram. Recognize that you are being asked to record the amount and not the dose.

Content Area: Child Health; **Category of Health Alteration:** Pharmacological and Parenteral Therapies; **Integrated Processes:** Nursing Process Implementation; **Client Need:** Physiological Integrity/Pharmacological and Parenteral Therapies/ Medication Administration; **Cognitive Level:** Analysis; **Reference:** Deglin, J., Vallerand, A., & Sanoski, C. (2011), p. 616.

261. A child who is having frequent, diarrheal stools is diagnosed with gastroenteritis and is hospitalized during a night shift. A health care provider (HCP) estimates the child lost 5% of the body weight due to severe diarrhea. At 0800 hours, an oncoming shift nurse reviews the child's medication administration record (MAR). Based on the MAR, which action should the nurse take **first**?

MEDICATION ADMINISTRATION RECORD

Date: Today

| Client Name: | Account Number: 23456 | Allergies: Ceftriaxone (Rocephin) |
| Date of Birth: 01-01-2007 | Weight: 20 kg | Dx: Gastroenteritis |

Medication	2400–0759	0800–1559	1600–2359
0.9% NaCl IV 50 mL/kg bolus infusion over 6 hours then discontinue	0200 NSN (1,000 mL at 166 mL/h)		
0.9% NaCl IV continuous maintenance infusion at 30 mL/hour after the bolus infusion is completed			
Acetaminophen (Tylenol) oral suspension 250 mg q4–6 h prn temp or pain	0300 NSN		
Diphenoxylate (Lomotil) oral suspension 2.5 mg/5 mL after each loose stool prn	0200 NSN (2.5 mg) 0500 NSN (2.5 mg) 0730 NSN (2.5 mg)		
Ampicillin sodium (Ampicin) 250 mg IV q6h	0200 NSN		
Signature: Night Shift Nurse, RN/NSN Day Shift Nurse, RN/DSN			

1. Assess the child's level of responsiveness.
2. Initiate the maintenance intravenous infusion after discontinuing the bolus infusion.
3. Assess the child for an allergic reaction to the first dose of ampicillin before administering the next dose.
4. Contact the HCP because the bolus infusion administered was the incorrect volume.

261. ANSWER: 1.

Diphenoxylate is a synthetic narcotic opiate agonist with central nervous system (CNS) side effects of sedation. The usual dose of diphenoxylate is 0.3–0.4 mg/kg/day of liquid in divided doses. For this child, the total daily dose is 6–8 mg. Within 5 ½ hours the child had received 7.5 mg of the 8 mg total daily dose. The bolus infusion should be completed at 0800 and the maintenance solution initiated, but this is not the first action. The child's reaction to ampicillin should be assessed before administering the dose of ampicillin that is due, but this is not the first action. The bolus infusion amount is correct. Fluid is administered to replace the deficit that has occurred. If 5% of the total weight is lost, then the fluid replacement is 50 mL/kg of body weight or 1,000 mL. The HCP should be contacted regarding the incomplete medication orders for diphenoxylate (Lomotil).

TEST-TAKING TIP: Read the situation and then read the options before reviewing the MAR. Consider side effects of medications and the nursing process steps.

Content Area: Child Health; **Category of Health Alteration:** Pharmacological and Parenteral Therapies; **Integrated Processes:** Nursing Process Analysis; **Client Need:** Physiological Integrity/Pharmacological and Parenteral Therapies/Adverse Effects/Contraindications/Interactions; **Cognitive Level:** Analysis; **Reference:** Wilson, B., Shannon, M., Shields, K., & Stang, C. (2008), pp. 91–92, 94–95, 278–279, 488–489.

262. A 3-year-old child with atopic dermatitis is prescribed to receive tacrolimus 0.03% (Protopic) topically to the affected area twice daily. Which instructions should a nurse include when teaching a parent? **Select all that apply.**

1. Apply a thin layer of ointment to the child's affected skin.
2. Use the ointment until the medication is gone.
3. Minimize your child's exposure to sunlight while using the ointment.
4. Apply the ointment after a bath while the skin is still wet.
5. Cover the medicated skin areas with an occlusive dressing.
6. Bring your child to the clinic after a week of medication for laboratory tests.

263. A nurse is conducting discharge planning for a child who will remain on oral digoxin (Lanoxin) therapy while at home. Which points are essential for the nurse to include in the teaching plan? **Select all that apply.**

1. Take the child's pulse for 1 minute prior to administration.
2. Adhere to the ordered laboratory testing.
3. Administer the medication with meals.
4. Notify the health care provider (HCP) if the child's pulse is less than 70 bpm.
5. Notify the HCP if the child has visual disturbances.
6. Administer digoxin immune fab (Digibind) if the child has overdosed on digoxin.

262. ANSWER: 1, 3.

Tacrolimus is absorbed into the skin; only a thin layer is needed. If exposed to ultraviolet light, the risk of skin cancer is increased. Natural and artificial sunlight should be avoided. Topical tacrolimus should be used until the symptoms are cleared and then discontinued. The skin should be clean and completely dry before application. The medicated skin area should be left uncovered.

TEST-TAKING TIP: Tacrolimus is a biological response modifier and immunosuppressant. Eliminate options that would enhance systemic absorption of the medication or increase the risk of cancer.

Content Area: Child Health; **Category of Health Alteration:** Pharmacological and Parenteral Therapies; **Integrated Processes:** Teaching and Learning; **Client Need:** Physiological Integrity/Pharmacological and Parenteral Therapies/Medication Administration; **Cognitive Level:** Application; **Reference:** Wilson, B., Shannon, M., Shields, K., & Stang, C. (2008), pp. 1442–1444.

263. ANSWER: 1, 2, 4, 5.

Digoxin should not be administered when the pulse is out of normal range, thus the pulse should be taken for a full minute prior to administration. The monitoring of laboratory specimens such as electrolyte and therapeutic drug levels are critical in avoiding toxicity or diminished efficacy. Although the literature suggests reporting a heart rate of less than 70 bpm for a child, the HCP should provide the child and parents with the range for the child and when to report a low value. Visual disturbances are a sign of digoxin toxicity. The drug should not be administered with food because this will delay absorption. Digibind is the antidote for digoxin toxicity, but the parents should not be instructed to administer this. Rather, the parents should be instructed to call 911.

Test-taking Tip: Applying basic knowledge of the pharmacological principles of digoxin would direct you to the correct responses. Eliminate option 3 because absorption is delayed and option 6 because the child's cardiac rhythm should be monitored.

Content Area: Child Health; **Category of Health Alteration:** Pharmacological and Parenteral Therapies; **Integrated Processes:** Teaching and Learning; **Client Need:** Physiological Integrity/Pharmacological and Parenteral Therapies/Medication Administration; **Cognitive Level:** Application; **References:** Berman, A., Snyder, S., Kozier, B., & Erb, G. (2008), p. 547; Deglin, J., & Vallerand, A. (2011), p. 439.

Tab 6 Psychosocial Integrity | Mental Health

Test 38: Mental Health: Anxiety and Mood Disorders

264. A nurse on the pediatric unit is caring for a 14-year-old girl who has frequent feelings of sadness. What factors should alert the nurse to possible depression that could lead to suicide? **Select all that apply.**

1. States sleeps 9 to 10 hours every night
2. Loss of interest in activities
3. Lack of school attendance
4. Previous suicide attempt
5. Desire to spend more time with friends than family
6. Frequent hospitalization

265. A nurse is teaching a class on strategies to cope with anxiety, using the technique of cognitive restructuring. To help a client develop these skills, prioritize the steps (1–4) that the nurse should teach the client.

_____ 1. Reflect by asking: "What is going on here? What am I thinking? Is the thought helpful?"

_____ 2. Stop. Break the cycle of negative thoughts.

_____ 3. Choose a more realistic, rational thought response.

_____ 4. Take a breath by eliciting a relaxation response and release tension.

264. ANSWER: 2, 3, 4, 6.
As depression increases there may be a loss of interest in activities and school attendance may drop. Once a client has attempted suicide, the client is at a greater risk to try again. Depression can affect every area of the body and therefore may trigger chronic illnesses and frequent hospitalizations. Many clients experiencing depression are unable to sleep soundly. An increased interest in spending time with friends is consistent with the developmental stage of a 14-year-old.

TEST-TAKING TIP: Apply knowledge of depression and suicide among adolescents to answer this question. Eliminate options 1 and 5 because these are consistent with the adolescent's developmental stage.

Content Area: Mental Health; **Category of Health Alteration:** Anxiety and Mood Disorders; **Integrated Processes:** Nursing Process Evaluation; **Client Need:** Psychosocial Integrity/Mental Health Concepts; **Cognitive Level:** Application; **Reference:** Ball, J., & Bindler, R. (2008), p. 1121.

265. ANSWER: 2, 4, 1, 3.
The nurse should first instruct the client to stop. This breaks the cycle of negative thoughts. Next, the client should be taught to take a breath by eliciting a relaxation response and release tension. Third, the client should reflect by asking: "What is going on here? What am I thinking? Is the thought helpful?" Finally, the client should choose a more realistic, rational thought response.

TEST-TAKING TIP: Anxiety situations can be exacerbated by negative, exaggerated thinking. Cognitive restructuring is a series of strategies that help clients evaluate their thoughts and replace them with more rational responses. Use this information to place the statements in the correct sequence.

Content Area: Mental Health; **Category of Health Alteration:** Anxiety and Mood Disorders; **Integrated Processes:** Teaching and Learning; **Client Need:** Physiological Integrity/Basic Care and Comfort/Nonpharmacological Comfort Interventions; **Cognitive Level:** Application; **References:** Edelman, C., & Mandle, C. (2006), pp. 300–301; Kneisl, C., & Trigoboff, E. (2009), pp. 461, 829–837.

266. A nurse assesses a client diagnosed with chronic lung disease who is receiving continuous home oxygen therapy. The client is apathetic and verbalizes very little during the assessment. Which additional assessment findings should the nurse associate with depression? **Select all that apply.**

1. Sleep disturbances
2. Confusion
3. Decreased appetite
4. Indecisiveness
5. Social withdrawal
6. Increased oxygen need from 2 to 3 liters

267. A client with treatment-resistant depression is being discharged from the mental health unit on vanlafaxine (Effexor). The client is to take 25 mg orally tid for 4 days, 50 mg orally tid for 4 days, and then 75 mg orally tid until the client's next office visit. The medication is supplied in 25-mg tablets. The nurse is explaining the medication regimen to the client and the client's spouse using a chart that lists the dates, dose, and number of tablets to be taken by the client. On the 10th day following discharge, how many tablets should the nurse instruct the client to take?

_____ tablets (Record your answer as a whole number.)

266. ANSWER: 1, 3, 4, 5.
The presence of sleep disturbances, decreased appetite, indecisiveness, and social withdrawal are behaviors observed in depression. Confusion or a decrease in level of responsiveness could be a sign of decreased brain oxygenation. A need to increase the oxygen concentration is more indicative of a worsening of the client's chronic lung disease.

TEST TAKING TIP: Eliminate any options that may indicate a worsening of the client's chronic lung disease.

Content Area: Mental Health; **Category of Health Alteration:** Anxiety and Mood Disorders; **Integrated Processes:** Nursing Process Assessment; **Client Need:** Psychosocial Integrity/Mental Health Concepts; **Cognitive Level:** Analysis; **References:** Ignatavicius, D., & Workman, M. (2010), pp. 628–635; Varcarolis, E., & Halter, M. (2009), pp. 221–222.

267. ANSWER: 3
If the client takes 25 mg for 4 days, then 50 mg for 4 days, on the 9th day after discharge the client should start taking 75 mg. If the medication is supplied in 25-mg tablets, the client should be taking three tablets three times daily on the 10th day following discharge.

TEST-TAKING TIP: Focus on what the question is asking. On the 9th day after discharge, the client should begin taking 75 mg and tablets are supplied in 25 mg.

Content Area: Mental Health; **Category of Health Alteration:** Anxiety and Mood Disorders; **Integrated Processes:** Teaching and Learning; **Client Need:** Health Promotion and Maintenance/Self-care; **Cognitive Level:** Analysis; **References:** Deglin, J., Vallerand, A., Danoski, C. (2011), p. 23; Varcarolis, E., & Halter, M. (2009), p. 235.

Test 39: Mental Health: Cognitive, Schizophrenic, and Psychotic Disorders

268. A home care nurse providing care for an 80-year-old male client diagnosed with Alzheimer's disease is assessing the home environment. The daughter who is the primary caregiver shares that she is getting very lonely and misses her own personal activities. Which responses by the nurse indicate appropriate nursing interventions in this situation? **Select all that apply.**

1. Suggesting she join an Alzheimer's support group
2. Praising her for "doing the right thing" for her father
3. Educating her to the signs and symptoms of depression
4. Exploring with her ways to interact with friends and family more
5. Explaining to her that her feelings of loneliness are normal and will pass
6. Identifying what aspect of caring for her father causes her to feel isolated

269. A client on the mental health unit is excessively agitated during the night shift. A nurse reviews the client's medication administration record (MAR). Based on the MAR, how many prn doses of alprazolam can the client receive within a 24-hour time period?

_____ prn doses (Record your answer as a whole number.)

MEDICATION ADMINISTRATION RECORD

Scheduled Medications	0001–0659	0700–1559	1600–2400
Alprazolam (Xanax) 1.5 mg orally tid		0800_____ 1400_____	2200_____
PRN Medications	0001–0659	0700–1559	1600–2400
Alprazolam (Xanax) 2.0 mg orally q4h prn (Do not exceed a total daily dose of 10 mg per day.)			

268. ANSWER: 1, 3, 4, 6.
Research has shown that full-time family caregivers report significantly higher levels of loneliness and depression than non-caregiving family members. Loneliness is a predictor of depression in such individuals. Identification of barriers to social interaction, therapeutic communication regarding feelings of isolation, and referral to support groups are all appropriate nursing interventions for this caregiving family member. Praise can cause feelings of guilt regarding feelings of loneliness and may curtail further discussion of the problem. Although feelings of loneliness may be normal for most caregivers, caregivers must address these feelings in order to prevent depression.

TEST-TAKING TIP: Use the process of elimination and focus on appropriate interventions directed toward self-management of the health and mental wellness of a caregiver.

Content Area: Mental Health; **Category of Health Alteration:** Cognitive, Schizophrenic, and Psychotic Disorders; **Integrated Process:** Nursing Process Implementation; **Client Needs:** Psychosocial Integrity/Mental Health Concepts; **Cognitive Ability:** Analysis; **Reference:** Varcarolis, E., & Halter, M. (2009), pp. 321, 476–477; **EBP Reference:** Family Caregiver Alliance. (2006). *Caregiver Assessment: Principles, Guidelines and Strategies for Change.* Report from a national consensus development conference (Volume I, p. 43). San Francisco: Family Caregiver Alliance. Retrieved from www.guideline.gov/summary/summary.aspx?doc_id=9670&nbr= 005179&string=alzheimer''s+AND+disease.

269. ANSWER: 2
The client can receive 2 prn doses within a 24-hour time period. The three times daily (tid) doses equal 4.5 mg ($1.5 \times 3 = 4.5$). If the maximum dose is 10 mg, then subtract 4.5 from 10 ($10 - 4.5 = 5.5$). The amount remaining is 5.5 mg. Next, the prn dose is 2 mg. Divide 5.5 by 2 ($5.5/2 = 2.75$). The number of doses remaining is 2. A partial dose of 0.75 mg cannot be given because the order is for 2 mg.

TEST-TAKING TIP: Be sure to consider that the maximum daily dose is 10 mg and that this includes the scheduled dose.

Content Area: Mental Health; **Category of Health Alteration:** Cognitive, Schizophrenic, and Psychotic Disorders; **Integrated Processes:** Nursing Process Analysis; **Client Need:** Physiological Integrity/Pharmacological and Parenteral Therapies/Dosage Calculation; **Cognitive Level:** Analysis; **References:** Deglin, J., & Vallerand, A. (2011), p. 138; Varcarolis, E., & Halter, M. (2009), p. 147.

270. A nurse manager reviewing documentation completed by a nurse working in a nursing home determines that the nurse needs additional instruction on caring for clients with acute confusion. Which chart documentation prompted the nurse manager's conclusion?

1. CLIENT A PROGRESS NOTES

Date	Time	Progress Notes
6-1-10	0900	Identification bracelet applied to client's wrist and updated picture taken for file records. K. Drew, R.N.

2. CLIENT B PROGRESS NOTES

Date	Time	Progress Notes
6-1-10	1000	Familiar belongings including pictures, cards, shawl, and purse placed in client's environment to reduce wandering behavior. _____K. Drew, R.N.

3. CLIENT C PROGRESS NOTES

Date	Time	Progress Notes
6-1-10	1100	Client reminded about why she is in the nursing home and redirected to the TV room after being found trying to exit from the visitor's entrance. _____K. Drew, R.N.

4. CLIENT D PROGRESS NOTES

Date	Time	Progress Notes
6-1-10	1300	Client allowed to wander in the nursing home garden. Made no attempts to venture beyond the garden gate. _____K. Drew, R.N.

270. ANSWER: 2.
A shawl and purse could be triggers and precipitate wandering activity. These should be removed from the client's view. A wristband and a recent photograph will aid in proper identification should the client wander. A client who wanders should be reassured in a calm, low-key voice tone about where the client is and why he or she is there and redirected to a safe environment. A reasonable amount of wandering in a safe, secure, designated environment, such as in the nursing home garden, may help to reduce the client's anxiety and frustration, provide physical exercise, improve cardiovascular function, and improve the client's self-esteem.

TEST-TAKING TIP: Consider the safety of the client and "triggers" that can increase wandering behavior.

Content Area: Mental Health; **Category of Health Alteration:** Cognitive, Schizophrenic, and Psychotic Disorders; **Integrated Processes:** Nursing Process Evaluation; **Client Need:** Safe and Effective Care Environment/Safety and Infection Control/Accident and Injury Prevention; **Cognitive Level:** Analysis; **References:** Fortinash, K., & Holoday Worret, P. (2007), p. 339; Townsend, M. (2009), p. 428.

271. A nurse is caring for a 30-year-old female with paranoid schizophrenia who was admitted 5 days ago to the mental health unit. The client's spouse is talking to the nurse after attending a family therapy session at the hospital. Which statements made by the client's spouse indicate that he needs **further education** on his wife's illness and management? **Select all that apply.**

1. "Food and fluids given to my wife should be in closed containers, such as a carton of yogurt."
2. "I plan on doing everything for my wife when she comes home so she can get better."
3. "Once at home, I should be discouraging visits from her friends for a while."
4. "I plan to ensure that she takes her prescribed medications so she won't experience a relapse."
5. "If my wife hallucinates, I should keep eye contact, call her by name, and speak simply but in a louder voice than usual."

271. ANSWER: 2, 3, 4.

Although tasks that require concentration and effort may be difficult for the client, especially during the acute phase of the illness, everything should not be done for the client by the spouse. Rather, her husband should encourage his wife to do things for herself with guidance. Visits from friends should not be discouraged but encouraged to minimize the risk for social isolation. Although relapses often occur due to nonadherence to the medication regimen, a relapse can occur while the client is taking medication. Relapses can be precipitated by stress and a lack of adaptive coping behaviors. Persons with paranoia might not eat or drink, thinking the food is poisoned. The client may perceive that food that hasn't been "tampered with" is safe to eat. Clients with paranoid schizophrenia experience delusions of persecution or grandeur and auditory hallucinations. The husband's response if his wife is hallucinating is appropriate.

TEST-TAKING TIP: The key phrase is "further education." Select options that discourage self-care and limits socialization. Consider that relapses can be precipitated by stress regardless of medication therapy.

Content Area: Mental Health; **Category of Health Alteration:** Cognitive, Schizophrenic, and Psychotic Disorders; **Integrated Process:** Teaching and Learning; **Client Needs:** Psychosocial Integrity/Mental Health Concepts; **Cognitive Ability:** Analysis; **Reference:** Varcarolis, E., & Halter, M. (2009), pp. 275–293.

272. A nurse is communicating with a client who is experiencing hallucinations. Which responses are most therapeutic? Place each response in numerical order (1–4) from the most therapeutic to the least therapeutic.

_____ 1. "If there were other voices I would hear them, too, wouldn't I?"

_____ 2. "The noise you hear is from the leaky faucet."

_____ 3. "The shadow is coming from the curtain. I will turn on the light so that you can see better."

_____ 4. "I don't see anything; tell me again what you think you see."

273. A nurse is attempting to deescalate the behavior of a client who has become violent and who is now placing an arm around another male client's neck. Which actions should the nurse take in this situation? **Select all that apply.**

1. Direct colleagues to move away from the client and the negotiating nurse.
2. Signal staff to call security and activate the assault team.
3. Move closer to the client and use gestures to get the client's attention.
4. Calmly state to the client, "The world seems terrible now, but you haven't done any harm to him."
5. Keep an open posture with the hands at the sides and palms outward.

272. ANSWER: 3, 2, 4, 1.
The responses from the most therapeutic to the least therapeutic are: "The shadow is coming from the curtain. I will turn on the light so that you can see better." "The noise you hear is from the leaky faucet." "I don't see anything; tell me again what you think you see." "If there were other voices I would hear them, too, wouldn't I?" The most therapeutic response promotes reality while offering a solution that helps enhance the client's senses. The next therapeutic response is one that promotes reality. It does not offer any solutions, however. The third option is challenging the client, but seeks clarification. The fourth option is nontherapeutic because it challenges the client.

TEST-TAKING TIP: The most therapeutic statement to a client who is hallucinating is one that promotes reality while offering solutions. A nontherapeutic response is one that challenges or contradicts the client. Use this information to place the statements in the correct sequence.

Content Area: Mental Health; **Category of Health Alteration:** Cognitive, Schizophrenic, and Psychotic Disorders; **Integrated Processes:** Communication and Documentation; **Client Need:** Psychosocial Integrity/Therapeutic Communications; **Cognitive Level:** Application; **References:** Fortinash, K., & Holoday Worret, P. (2007), p. 342. Townsend, M. (2009), pp. 132–134.

273. ANSWER: 2, 4, 5.
Calling security and the assault team will protect the client and others from harm or injury as a result of a possible lethal attack. Communicating in a calm voice and reminding the client that he has not yet harmed anyone, shows empathy and encourages cooperation. It shows that the nurse is listening. An open posture sends a nonthreatening message and a willingness to listen. Another colleague should stay nearby the nurse for protection. Moving closer than about 8 feet and using gestures can escalate the aggressive behavior.

TEST-TAKING TIP: Consider the nurse's safety and eliminate options that increase the nurse's risk of harm.

Content Area: Mental Health; **Category of Health Alteration:** Cognitive, Schizophrenic, and Psychotic Disorders; **Integrated Processes:** Nursing Process Implementation; **Client Need:** Psychosocial Integrity/Mental Health Concepts; **Cognitive Level:** Application; **Reference:** Fortinash, K., & Holoday Worret, P. (2008), pp. 278–279.

Test 40: Mental Health: Crisis, Violence, Eating, and Sleep Disorders

274. A nurse is planning a staff development program on the care of clients diagnosed with a post-traumatic stress disorder (PTSD). Which information should the nurse include in the program? **Select all that apply.**

1. Migraine headaches can really impact the life of a client diagnosed with PTSD.
2. Clients diagnosed with PTSD require regular assessment for signs of depression.
3. Unrealistic fears are a common physical outcome of persons diagnosed with PTSD.
4. Some clients with PTSD experience survivor guilt if others died in the traumatic event.
5. A diagnosis of PTSD is made based on the symptoms that occur within the first few days after the traumatic event.

275. A nurse is interviewing parents during their 5-year-old daughter's admission to a hospital. The child is admitted for a broken arm and cuts on her abdomen. Which observations should alert the nurse to abuse? **Select all that apply.**

1. The parents are showing concern for their child.
2. The parents lack ability to comfort their child.
3. The parents do not seem to understand how their child may be feeling.
4. The parents maintain the child is responsible for the injuries.
5. The parents act as if the injury is an assault on them.

274. ANSWER: 1, 2, 3, 4.

Migraines, symptoms of depression, unrealistic fears, and survivor guilt are all associated with PTSD. Diagnostic criteria for PTSD include a duration of the disturbance for more than 1 month and is not based on symptoms occurring within the first few days after the traumatic event. Symptoms may appear within the first 3 months after the trauma or be delayed for months or years.

TEST-TAKING TIP: Note that four options are similar and one is different. Eliminate the option that is different from the others.

Content Area: Mental Health; **Category of Health Alteration:** Crisis, Violence, Eating, and Sleep Disorders; **Integrated Processes:** Nursing Process Planning; **Client Need:** Psychosocial Integrity/Crisis Intervention; **Cognitive Level:** Analysis; **Reference:** Townsend, M. (2008), pp. 398–399.

275. ANSWER: 2, 3, 4, 5.

Parents who abuse their children often seem to show no ability to comfort or understand their child. The parents maintain that the child is responsible for the injury, such as the child fell or the child cut herself. Parents who abuse children may seem to act as if they are the victims. Abusive parents do not tend to show concern for their child. However, this may be difficult to determine and identify.

TEST-TAKING TIP: Select the options that place the focus on the parents and not on the child.

Content Area: Mental Health/Child Health; **Category of Health Alteration:** Crisis, Violence, Eating, and Sleep Disorders; **Integrated Processes:** Nursing Process Assessment; **Client Need:** Psychosocial Integrity/Abuse/Neglect; **Cognitive Level:** Analysis; **Reference:** Ball, J., & Binder, R. (2008), pp. 240–241.

276. An older adult client with a forehead laceration is admitted to the emergency department accompanied by his daughter with whom he resides. The client has poor eye contact and looks to his daughter for answers as to the nature of his injury. On observation, the client is noted to have scattered bruises and welt marks. Which questions should the nurse ask during the assessment of the client after the daughter leaves the room? **Select all that apply.**

1. "Are you satisfied living with your daughter?"
2. "Do you have the finances to be able to pay for your health care?"
3. "Have you been drinking more alcoholic beverages lately?"
4. "Has anyone ever hurt you?"
5. "Can you tell me more about how your injury occurred?"

277. A nurse is reviewing the assessment findings of a 76-year-old client receiving haloperidol (Haldol). Which conclusions should the nurse make based on the findings? **Select all that apply.**

PHYSICAL FINDINGS

Neurological	Tremor, slurred speech, dystonia, akathisia
Ears	Presbycusis, increased ear wax secretion
Musculoskeletal system	Bone calcification, lordosis
Integument	Increased facial hair and moist, supple skin

1. The client is experiencing extra-pyramidal side effects from the medication.
2. The client is showing side effects from the medication in all the body systems noted.
3. Presbycusis and increased earwax secretion are age-related changes.
4. Bone calcification and lordosis are age-related changes.
5. Increased facial hair and moist, supple skin are normal findings.

276. ANSWER: 1, 4, 5.

Indicators of potential physical abuse include laceration, poor eye contact, looks to daughter for answers, bruises, and welt marks. Asking questions further assesses for abuse and ascertains the client's physical safety. The client's responses about his satisfaction with living arrangements, ever being hurt by another, or the nature of the current injury will provide further information to evaluate whether abuse is occurring. The client may be reluctant to talk about the abuse due to shame, self-blame, abandonment, or further mistreatment. Asking a question about the client's financial situation is inappropriate. To evaluate for financial exploitation, the nurse should ask who manages the client's finances. There is no indication that the client consumes alcohol.

TEST-TAKING TIP: Focus on questions that pertain to the client's physical safety and eliminate the other options.

Content Area: Mental Health; **Category of Health Alteration:** Crisis, Violence, Eating, and Sleep Disorders; **Integrated Processes:** Nursing Process Assessment; **Client Need:** Psychosocial Integrity/Abuse/Neglect; **Cognitive Level:** Application; **Reference:** Fortinash, K., & Holoday Worret, P. (2008), p. 502.

277. ANSWER: 1, 3.

Extra-pyramidal side effects include tremor, slurred speech, dystonia, and akathisia. Presbycusis (loss of acuity for high-frequency tones) and an increase in earwax secretion are normal age-related changes. Only the CNS is showing side effects of haloperidol use, not all systems. Bone calcification and lordosis are abnormal, but these are not related to the medication or the client's age. Increased facial hair and moist supple skin are not normal for an older adult. Decreased (not increased) facial hair in men is a normal age-related change. The skin is usually dry but with care can be moist and supple.

TEST-TAKING TIP: Examine each option carefully. Select options focusing on both the side effects of the medication and the client's age.

Content Area: Mental Health; **Category of Health Alteration:** Crisis, Violence, Eating, and Sleep Disorders; **Integrated Processes:** Nursing Process Evaluation; **Client Need:** Physiological Integrity/Pharmacological and Parenteral Therapies/ Adverse Effects/Contraindications/Interactions; **Cognitive Level:** Analysis; **References:** Potter, P., & Perry, A. (2009), pp. 198–201; Wilson, B., Shannon, M., Shields, K., & Stang, C. (2008), pp. 727–729.

Test 41: Mental Health: End-of-Life Care

278. A 20-year-old client has just died as a result of an automobile accident, and nurses present in the emergency department are supporting family members. Which statements made by a nurse are supportive? **Select all that apply.**

1. "I am so sorry for your loss."
2. "It's God will that he should die so young."
3. "It will get better with time."
4. "You still have your other son, who survived the accident."
5. "Do you wish to spend time alone with your son? I can arrange this for you."
6. "You can stay as long as you would like to be with your son. Is there anything I can do for you?"

279. An elderly woman is receiving palliative care at her daughter's home. The daughter is her mother's caregiver. The client has had several strokes, is unable to speak, and can move only her left-sided extremities. The daughter tells a nurse that she is concerned that her mother is in pain at times and cannot communicate her distress. Which behaviors associated with pain should the nurse teach the daughter to recognize? **Select all that apply.**

1. Restlessness
2. Resisting turning or positioning
3. Relaxed facial expression
4. Tense muscles
5. Crying or moaning
6. Guarding a painful body area with her left upper extremities

278. ANSWER: 1, 5, 6.

Statements 1, 5, and 6 are supportive statements. A simple statement expressing sympathy is best. Family may wish to be alone with the body but may be afraid to ask. **The body should never be removed until the family is ready.** Option 2 is making a statement that interprets the situation for the family, which should be avoided. Options 3 and 4 are making statements that mitigate the family's grief and are not supportive.

TEST-TAKING TIP: The key word is "supportive." Eliminate options that interpret the situation or mitigate the family's grief.

Content Area: Mental Health; **Category of Health Alteration:** End-of-Life Care; **Integrated Processes:** Communication and Documentation; **Client Need:** Psychosocial Integrity/Grief and Loss; **Cognitive Level:** Analysis; **Reference:** Wilkinson, J., & Treas, L. (2011), pp. 162–163.

279. ANSWER: 1, 2, 4, 5, 6.

Nonverbal behaviors associated with stress, protecting a body area by resisting movement or guarding, and vocalizing discomfort can all indicate pain. A relaxed facial expression is associated with comfort.

TEST-TAKING TIP: Read the scenario in the stem carefully. The issue of the question is recognition of pain in clients who cannot speak. Evaluate each option and select those associated with expression of pain.

Content Area: Mental Health; **Category of Health Alteration:** End-of-Life Care; **Integrated Processes:** Analysis; **Client Need:** Psychosocial Integrity/Sensory/Perceptual Alterations; **Cognitive Level:** Application; **Reference:** Berman, A., Snyder, S., Kozier, B., & Erb, G. (2008), p. 1096.

280. A nurse notes that an older adult client who is dying is becoming more anxious due to increasing dyspnea and fear of suffocation. Which nursing actions would be appropriate when caring for the client? **Select all that apply.**

1. Turn off the fan at the client's bedside.
2. Elevate the head of the bed (HOB) 30–45 degrees.
3. Administer oxygen at 2 liters per nasal cannula.
4. Administer lorazepam (Ativan) 0.5–1 mg IV q4–6h prn.
5. Administer morphine sulfate 2.5 mg orally q4h prn.

281. A nurse is caring for a 4-year-old Chinese American client of the Buddhist faith who just died. Which behaviors exhibited by those in the room would be characteristic of the client's religious beliefs and customs? **Select all that apply.**

1. Family members are avoiding eye contact with the nurse when listening.
2. A family member requests a rabbi's presence.
3. Black armbands are worn around the upper arms of those present.
4. A white strip of cloth is tied around the heads of those present.
5. A family member asks to place a dish of tobacco near the client's bedside.
6. Family members are all crying and hugging each other and the nurses.

280. ANSWER: 2, 3, 4, 5.
Elevating the head of the bed reduces oxygen consumption and promotes maximal lung expansion. Oxygen may decrease hypoxemia or it may have a placebo effect and decrease anxiety. Lorazepam is an anti-anxiety medication used to reduce restlessness and decrease respiratory effort. Morphine reduces the excessive respiratory drive caused by anxiety and hypoxemia, slows ventilation, and makes breathing more effective. The fan should be left turned on because air movement provides a sense that more oxygen is available and decreases the feelings of suffocation.

TEST-TAKING TIP: Note the key words "anxious" and "dyspnea." Select interventions to treat both problems.

Content Area: Mental Health; **Category of Health Alteration:** End-of-Life Care; **Integrated Processes:** Nursing Process Implementation; **Client Need:** Physiological Integrity/Physiological Adaptation/Alterations in Body Systems; **Cognitive Level:** Application; **Reference:** Mauk, K. (2010), pp. 61–62.

281. ANSWER: 1, 3, 4.
The Chinese avoid direct eye contact when listening. Mourners wear black armbands and white strips of cloth tied around their heads. For those of Chinese American descent, white is associated with death. A family of the Jewish, not the Buddhist, faith would request a rabbi's presence. Tobacco is important in Native American rituals. The Chinese often do not express their emotions openly and they prefer not to be touched by strangers.

TEST-TAKING TIP: Focus on the client's religious belief and ethnic background. Recall that Chinese Americans associate black with bad luck and white with death.

Content Area: Mental Health; **Category of Health Alteration:** End-of-Life Care; **Integrated Processes:** Caring; **Client Need:** Psychosocial Integrity/Religious and Spiritual Influences on Health; **Cognitive Level:** Application; **References:** Ball, J., & Bindler, R. (2008), pp. 149, 462; Harkreader, H., Hogan, M., & Thobaben, M. (2007), pp. 54–57; Townsend, M. (2008), pp. 650–652.

Test 42: Mental Health: Personality Disorders

282. A nurse educator orienting new nurses is discussing borderline personality disorders. The nurse educator states that individuals with borderline personality disorder exhibit affective instability, transient psychotic episodes, and impulsive, aggressive, and suicidal behavior. When showing an illustration of the brain, which area should the nurse identify as causing the behaviors of anxiety, rage, and fear? Mark the affected area with an X.

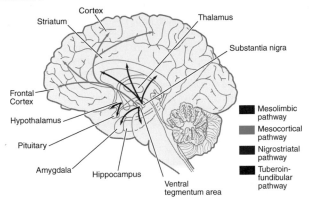

282. ANSWER:

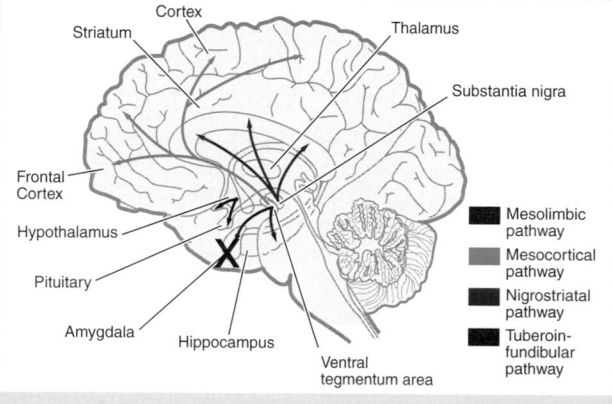

The amygdala is associated with anxiety, rage, and fear. Studies have shown a decrease in serotonin activity and an increase in alpha-2 norandrenergic receptor sites may be related to the irritability and impulsiveness common to people with borderline personality disorder. An increase in dopamine may be responsible for transient psychotic states. The limbic structures are associated with emotional alterations and the prefrontal and frontal cortices control modulation of social judgment.

TEST-TAKING TIP: A memory cue is to associate the "a" in anxiety with the "a" in <u>a</u>mygdala. It is necessary to be familiar with brain structures and the areas responsible for behaviors and emotion.

Content Area: Mental Health; **Category of Health Alteration:** Personality Disorders; **Integrated Processes:** Teaching and Learning; **Client Need:** Psychosocial Integrity/Mental Health Concepts; **Cognitive Level:** Application; **Reference:** Boyd, M. (2008), p. 443.

283. A nurse is counseling a client with passive-aggressive disorder. Which roles might a nurse observe displayed by the client? **Select all that apply.**

1. The martyr
2. The misunderstood
3. The contrite
4. The guilt-ridden
5. The sickly individual
6. The individual with an IQ of 60

284. A nurse caring for a client with antisocial personality disorder writes the following nursing diagnosis in the client's care plan: "Defensive coping related to dysfunctional family system as evidenced by disregard for laws, absence of guilty feelings, and inability to delay gratification." Which interventions should the nurse include for this client? **Select all that apply.**

1. Provide positive feedback for acceptable behavior.
2. Have sufficient staff available to present a show of strength to the client.
3. Convince the client to do what is right by using the words "You should . . . ."
4. Administer consequences immediately following an infraction of a unit rule.
5. Lengthen the time requirement to receive a reward for acceptable behavior.

283. ANSWER: 1, 2, 3, 4, 5.

Passive-aggressive individuals are prone to playing multiple roles depending on the circumstances. Passive-aggressive individuals are unable to express their anger directly. They may appear polite and helpful, but they express their anger and hostility in subtle ways. Playing these roles is a tactic used to demonstrate anger and resentment while gaining dependency, attention, and reassurance. An IQ of 60 indicates mental retardation. This is not a role that would be assumed.

TEST-TAKING TIP: Visualize each option to determine whether the option is a role that can be assumed by a person with passive-aggressive disorder. Eliminate option 6 because it is different from the others.

Content Area: Mental Health; **Category of Health Alteration:** Personality Disorders; **Integrated Process:** Nursing Process Analysis; **Client Need:** Psychosocial Integrity/ Coping Mechanisms; **Cognitive Level:** Analysis; **Reference:** Townsend, M. (2008), pp. 503–504.

284. ANSWER: 1, 4, 5.

Positive reinforcement enhances the client's self-esteem and encourages repeating desirable behaviors. Undesirable consequences may help to decrease repeating undesirable behaviors. Lengthening the time required to receive a reward may assist the client in learning to delay gratification. Presenting a show of strength with multiple staff is an intervention for risk in other-directed violence. Attempts should not be made to coax or convince the client to do the "right thing," using words such as "You should . . . ." The phrase "You will be expected to . . ." should be used instead.

TEST-TAKING TIP: Eliminate options that do not pertain to the information provided in the nursing diagnosis. Remember, explanations to the client must be concrete and clear.

Content Area: Mental Health; **Category of Health Alteration:** Personality Disorders; **Integrated Processes:** Nursing Process Analysis; **Client Need:** Safe and Effective Care Environment/Management of Care/Continuity of Care; **Cognitive Level:** Analysis; **Reference:** Townsend, M. (2008), pp. 514–515.

285. A mental health unit is using assessment, problem, intervention, and evaluation (APIE) method of documentation. An experienced nurse is reviewing documentation completed by a new nurse and finds the documentation in the incorrect order. When instructing the new nurse on the correct order for documentation, in which order should the experienced nurse place the information? Place the nurse's documentation in the correct order (1–4) using the APIE documentation method.

_____ 1. Initiated trusting relationship by spending time alone with the client. Discussed his feelings regarding interactions with others and accompanied client to group activities. Provided positive feedback for voluntarily participating in assertiveness training.

_____ 2. Social isolation related to inability to trust, panic level of anxiety, and delusional thinking.

_____ 3. Client states he does not want to sit with or talk to others; they "frighten" him. Stays in room unless strongly encouraged to come out. No group involvement. At times listens to group conversations from a distance but does not interact; some hypervigilance and scanning noted.

_____ 4. Cooperative with therapy but still uncomfortable in the presence of a group of people. Accepted nurse's positive feedback.

286. A client with avoidant personality disorder is started on paroxetine (Paxil) after a panic disorder developed. Which findings on assessment should prompt a nurse to consider that the client is experiencing adverse effects from the medication? **Select all that apply.**

1. Urinary frequency
2. Tremor
3. Taste aversion
4. Excess salivation
5. Sedation

285. ANSWER: 3, 2, 1, 4.
The assessment should be first: Client states he does not want to sit with or talk to others; they "frighten" him. Stays in room unless strongly encouraged to come out. No group involvement. At times listens to group conversations from a distance but does not interact; some hypervigilance and scanning noted. The problem should be second: Social isolation related to inability to trust, panic level of anxiety, and delusional thinking. The intervention should be third: Initiated trusting relationship by spending time alone with the client. Discussed his feelings regarding interactions with others and accompanied client to group activities. Provided positive feedback for voluntarily participating in assertiveness training. The evaluation is fourth: Cooperative with therapy but still uncomfortable in the presence of a group of people. Accepted nurse's positive feedback.

TEST-TAKING TIP: Use the acronym APIE to place the statements in the correct sequence.

Content Area: Mental Health; **Category of Health Alteration:** Personality Disorders; **Integrated Processes:** Communication and Documentation; **Client Need:** Psychosocial Integrity/Mental Health Concepts; **Cognitive Level:** Application; **Reference:** Townsend, M. (2008), pp. 135–136.

286. ANSWER: 1, 2, 3, 5.
Urinary frequency, tremor, taste aversion, and sedation are all adverse effects of paroxetine. Dry mouth, not excess salivation, is also an adverse effect.

TEST-TAKING TIP: Eliminate the one option that is opposite of an adverse effect.

Content Area: Mental Health; **Category of Health Alteration:** Personality Disorders; **Integrated Processes:** Nursing Process Evaluation; **Client Need:** Physiological Integrity/Pharmacological and Parenteral Therapies/Adverse Effects/Contraindications/Interactions; **Cognitive Level:** Application; **Reference:** Wilson, B., Shannon, M., Shields, K., & Stang, C. (2008), pp. 1161–1163.

Test 43: Mental Health: Substance Abuse

287. Six months after being started on disulfiram (Antabuse) for treatment of alcoholism, a 58-year-old male client has serum laboratory tests completed. Which findings on the client's laboratory report should prompt a nurse to immediately notify the health care provider (HCP) of the results? Place an X in the blank space next to the laboratory value results for the findings that should be reported immediately to the HCP.

Serum Laboratory Test	Client's Value
Potassium	4.0 mEq/L
Red blood cells	4.9 m/mm³
Hemoglobin	12 g/dL
Albumin	2.8 g/dL
AST	65 units/L
ALT	60 units/L
Total bilirubin	3.8 mg/dL
ALP	160 units/L

288. A roommate brings a college student with a history of drug abuse to the clinic because of suspected barbiturate overdose. Which assessment findings should the nurse associate with the barbiturate overdose? **Select all that apply.**

1. Watery eyes
2. Nasal stuffiness
3. Shallow respirations
4. Weak, rapid pulse
5. Decreased blood pressure

287. ANSWER:

The liver enzymes are abnormal. When taking disulfiram, liver function tests (LFTs) are drawn initially, then at 10–14 days, and then every 6 months thereafter. The chart below shows the normal values.

Serum Laboratory Test and Normal Values	Client's Value	
Albumin (3.2–4.6 g/dL)	2.8 g/dL	X
Aspartate aminotransferase (AST) (15–40 units/L)	65 units/L	X
Alanine aminotransferase (ALT) (10–40 units/L)	60 units/L	X
Total bilirubin (0.2–1.3 mg/dL)	3.8 mg/dL	X
Alkaline phospatase (ALP) (35–142 units/L)	160 units/L	X

TEST-TAKING TIP: A method for remembering the LFTs is to think of Alcoholics Anonymous (AA) and use the AA as a memory cue for the four LFTs that begin with the letter A (albumin, AST, ALT, ALP). Then recall that there are five LFTs and that the letter B follows A to remember bilirubin.

Content Area: Mental Health; **Category of Health Alteration:** Substance Abuse; **Integrated Processes:** Nursing Process Analysis; **Client Need:** Physiological Integrity/Reduction of Risk Potential/Laboratory Values; **Cognitive Level:** Analysis; **References:** Van Leeuwen, A., & Poelhuis-Leth, D. (2009), pp. 13, 15, 23, 159; Varcarolis, E., & Halter, M. (2009), p. 355.

288. ANSWER: 3, 4, 5.

The central nervous system effects of a barbiturate overdose are shallow respirations, weak and rapid pulse, and decreased blood pressure. Watery eyes and nasal stuffiness are not signs of an overdose from barbiturates.

TEST-TAKING TIP: Select options that relate to acute respiratory and cardiovascular effects.

Content Area: Mental Health; **Category of Health Alteration:** Substance Abuse; **Integrated Processes:** Nursing Process Assessment; **Client Need:** Psychosocial Integrity/Chemical and Other Dependencies; **Cognitive Level:** Application; **Reference:** Varcarolis, E., & Halter, M. (2009), p. 341.

289. A client is brought to the emergency department after overdosing on lorazepam (Ativan). Which actions should the nurse take when caring for this client? **Select all that apply.**

1. Administer activated charcoal.
2. Check vital signs every 15 minutes.
3. Initiate an intravenous access.
4. Pad side rails.
5. Administer naloxone hydrochloride (Narcan).
6. Place on a cooling blanket.

290. A nurse is using the CAGE-AID Screening Tool to screen a client for alcohol and substance abuse. If used according to the acronym, in which order should the nurse ask the client the questions on the tool? Place each question in the correct numerical order (1–4) for using the CAGE-AID Screening Tool.

_____ 1. Have you ever had a drink (used drugs) first thing in the morning (eye-opener) to steady your nerves or get rid of a hangover?
_____ 2. Have people annoyed you by criticizing your drinking (drug use)?
_____ 3. Have you ever felt you ought to cut down on your drinking (or drug use)?
_____ 4. Have you ever felt bad or guilty about your drinking (drug use)?

289. ANSWER: 1, 2, 3, 4.
Activated charcoal is administered to aid absorption of the drug. Drug overdose produces shock; monitoring vital signs every 15 minutes alerts the nurse to a change in the client's status. An intravenous access is needed for administering emergency medications. Seizures can occur from the overdose effects of lorazepam; precautions are necessary for preventing injury to the client. Naloxone is a narcotic antagonist, administered for an opiate overdose. Rather, flumazenil (Romazicon), a benzodiazepine antagonist, should be administered. Hyperpyrexia is not an overdose effect from lorazepam.

TEST-TAKING TIP: Lorazepam is a benzodiazepine. Eliminate any options that pertain to an opiate overdose and not benzodiazepine overdose.

Content Area: Mental Health; **Category of Health Alteration:** Substance Abuse; **Integrated Processes:** Nursing Process Implementation; **Client Need:** Physiological Integrity/Physiological Adaptation/Medical Emergencies; **Cognitive Level:** Analysis; **Reference:** Varcarolis, E., & Halter, M. (2009), pp. 341, 345.

290. ANSWER: 3, 2, 4, 1.
Key words in the questions correspond to the acronym. The first key word is "cut" making this question first: "Have you ever felt you ought to cut down on your drinking (or drug use)?" The second key word is "annoyed," making this question second: "Have people annoyed you by criticizing your drinking (drug use)?" The third key word is "guilty" making this question third: "Have you ever felt bad or guilty about your drinking (drug use)?" The last key word is "eye-opener," making this question fourth: "Have you ever had a drink (used drugs) first thing in the morning (eye-opener) to steady your nerves or get rid of a hangover?"

TEST-TAKING TIP: Look for key words in the questions that correspond to the acronym of CAGE.

Content Area: Mental Health; **Category of Health Alteration:** Substance Abuse; **Integrated Processes:** Nursing Process Assessment; **Client Need:** Psychosocial Integrity/Chemical and other Dependencies; **Cognitive Level:** Application; **Reference:** Varcarolis, E., & Halter, M. (2009), p. 340.

Test 44: Mental Health: Pharmacological and Parenteral Therapies

291. A nurse is to administer haloperidol (Haldol) 2 mg IV now to a client in acute psychosis. A vial of haloperidol 5 mg/mL is available. How many milliliters of medication should the nurse administer?

_____ mL (Record your answer to the nearest tenth.)

292. A nurse is caring for a hospitalized client who begins to develop delirium tremens (DTs). After notifying the health care provider (HCP), which interventions should the nurse expect to include when caring for this client? **Select all that apply.**

1. Administer vitamin therapy.
2. Provide reality orientation.
3. Confront the client when hallucinating.
4. Encourage visits from family members.
5. Administer benzodiazepines, such as lorazepam (Ativan).

291. ANSWER: 0.4

Use a proportion formula to calculate the dose. Then multiply the extremes (outside values) and means (inside values) to solve for *X*.

5 mg : 1 mL :: 2 mg : *X* mL

$5X = 2$

$X = 0.4$

TEST-TAKING TIP: If the dose obtained is 1 or more, then check your calculations.

Content Area: Mental Health; **Category of Health Alteration:** Pharmacological and Parenteral Therapies; **Integrated Processes:** Nursing Process Implementation; **Client Need:** Physiological Integrity/Pharmacological and Parenteral Therapies/ Dosage Calculation; **Cognitive Level:** Application; **Reference:** Pickar, G., & Abernethy, A. (2008), p. 46.

292. ANSWER: 1, 2, 5.

Vitamins, such as B vitamins, help to calm the agitated central nervous system and prevent anemia and peripheral neuropathy. Reality orientation helps to reduce fear and confusion. Benzodiazepines are administered to decrease seizures. If hallucinating, an intervention should present a nonthreatening reality to the client rather than confront the client, which could increase the client's agitation and lead to injury. Stimulation should be reduced, not increased.

TEST-TAKING TIP: Focus on the fact that the nurse is notifying the HCP. Select collaborative interventions.

Content Area: Mental Health; **Category of Health Alteration:** Pharmacological and Parenteral Therapies; **Integrated Processes:** Nursing Process Planning; **Client Need:** Psychosocial Integrity/Chemical and other Dependencies; **Cognitive Level:** Application; **References:** Fortinash, K., & Holoday Worret, P. (2007), pp. 389–394; Ignatavicius, D., & Workman, M. (2010), p. 84.

293. A client has a transdermal patch of selegiline (EMSAM). During a clinic visit the client shows a nurse a list of prohibited foods. The client's daughter created the list based on the foods and beverages the client likes to eat but now avoids due to the medication. When examining the list, which foods should the nurse question whether these are prohibited for another reason? Place an X in the blank space next to the foods about which the nurse should question the client further.

Prohibited Foods
Aged cheeses
Ripe avocados
Kiwi
Liver
Pickled herring
Strawberries
Chianti and sherry
Delicatessen meats
Sausage
Shrimp

294. A client calls the clinic to tell the nurse that the client's depression has not improved after 1 week of amitriptyline (Elavil). Which responses by the nurse are appropriate? **Select all that apply.**

1. "Have you noticed a decrease in your anxiety or any improvement in sleep?"
2. "I will inform the health care provider (HCP) who can prescribe a stronger medication."
3. "It may be necessary to increase your medication dose."
4. "Have you become more involved in activities since beginning the medication?"
5. "It usually takes 2 to 4 weeks to see a relief of your depressed mood."

293. ANSWER:

Kiwi	X
Strawberries	X
Shrimp	X

Kiwi, strawberries, and shrimp are not prohibited for a client taking selegiline, a monamine oxidase inhibitor (MAOI). Foods high in tyramine content such as aged cheeses, raisins, red wines, smoked and processed meats, pickled herring, meat tenderizer, and soy sauce, should be avoided while on MAOIs. Persons with allergies are often allergic to kiwi, strawberries, and shrimp.

TEST-TAKING TIP: Identify the foods that often cause allergic reactions. Remember that those with an allergy to kiwi often have a latex allergy. Eliminate foods high in tyramine because these should be avoided when taking MAOIs.

Content Area: Mental Health; **Category of Health Alteration:** Pharmacological and Parenteral Therapies; **Integrated Processes:** Nursing Process Analysis; **Client Need:** Physiological Integrity/Pharmacological and Parenteral Therapies/Adverse Effects/Contraindications/Interactions; **Cognitive Level:** Analysis; **Reference:** Fortinash, K., & Holoday Worret, P. (2008), pp. 553–556.

294. ANSWER: 1, 4, 5.
Effects usually seen in the first week include decreased anxiety and improved sleep, but clients are often unaware of these changes. An increase in activity indicates a positive response to therapy and usually occurs in 1 to 3 weeks. It takes 2 to 4 weeks to achieve relief of the depressed mood. It is premature to recommend a stronger medication or to increase the dose.

TEST-TAKING TIP: Use the nursing process to select options that collect additional information. Eliminate options that take an action without further assessment.

Content Area: Mental Health; **Category of Health Alteration:** Pharmacological and Parenteral Therapies; **Integrated Processes:** Nursing Process Assessment; **Client Need:** Physiological Integrity/Pharmacological and Parenteral Therapies/Expected Actions or Outcomes; **Cognitive Level:** Analysis; **Reference:** Fortinash, K., & Holoday Worret, P. (2008), p. 555.

295. During an office visit, a nurse questions a client whose medication was changed from the benzodiazepine, temazepam (Restoril), to zolpidem (Ambien CR) due to experiencing side effects from the temazepam. Which questions would be most helpful to ask the client to determine if the change in medication was advantageous? **Select all that apply.**

1. "Are there some nights that you do not need to take zolpidem for sleep?"
2. "Do you notice a reduction in your anxiety now that you started the zolpidem?"
3. "Are you able to fall asleep and stay asleep every night since beginning zolpidem?"
4. "Are you having any stomach upset now that you can take zolpidem with food?"
5. "Have you had any hallucinations since starting zolpidem?"

296. A nurse is to administer a total of 300 mg of desipramine (Norpramin) daily in two divided doses to a client with major depression. The desipramine is supplied in 100-mg tablets. How many tablets should the nurse administer with each dose?

_____tablets (Record your answer to the nearest tenth.)

295. ANSWER: 1, 3.

Advantages of nonbenzodiazepine hypnotics, such as zolpidem, over benzodiazepines include avoidance of dependence and lack of rebound insomnia. Zolpidem possesses minimal anxiolytic properties; this is not an advantage over temazepam. Zolpidem should be taken on an empty stomach because food decreases absorption. A side effect of zolpidem is hallucinations.

TEST-TAKING TIP: The key word is "advantageous." Select the questions that focus on the advantages of a nonbenzodiazepine over a benzodiazepine. Consider the side effects of both.

Content Area: Mental Health; **Category of Health Alteration:** Pharmacological and Parenteral Therapies; **Integrated Processes:** Nursing Process Evaluation; **Client Need:** Physiological Integrity/Pharmacological and Parenteral Therapies/ Expected Actions or Outcomes; **Cognitive Level:** Analysis; **Reference:** Fortinash, K., & Holoday Worret, P. (2008), p. 567.

296. ANSWER: 1.5

Use a proportion formulation to calculate the dose. Then, multiply the extremes (outside values) and means (inside values) to solve for X.

100 mg : 1 tab :: 300 mg : X tabs

100 X = 300

X = 3 tabs total daily dose

Then divide the total daily dose of 3 tabs by 2 to administer a total of 1.5 tabs with each dose.

TEST-TAKING TIP: Focus on the information in the question. During the actual NCLEX-RN, use the on-screen calculator if needed. Verify your answer, especially if it seems like an unusual amount. Key word phrase is "*each* dose."

Content Area: Mental Health; **Category of Health Alteration:** Pharmacological and Parenteral Therapies; **Integrated Processes:** Nursing Process Implementation; **Client Need:** Physiological Integrity/Pharmacological and Parenteral Therapies/ Dosage Calculation; **Cognitive Level:** Application; **Reference:** Pickar, G., & Abernethy, A. (2008), p. 46.

297. When assessing a client taking oxcarbazepine (Trileptal) for treatment of acute bipolar mania, a nurse concludes that the client is experiencing signs of carbamazepine toxicity and notifies the health care provider (HCP). Which observations prompted the nurse's action? **Select all that apply.**

1. Excessive salivation
2. Ataxia
3. Sedation
4. Diplopia
5. Agitation
6. Dizziness

298. A client with bipolar mania is receiving olanzapine (Zyprexa). A nurse caring for the client on the mental health unit documents in the client's medical record. An oncoming shift nurse reviews the previous nurse's documentation. Which conclusion by the oncoming shift nurse is correct?

PROGRESS NOTES

Date	Time	Progress Notes
Today	1300	Excessively restless today with pacing, rocking, and inability to sit still. Much lip smacking and writhing movements of the fingers and toes noted. Easily distracted, going from one action to the next. Making numerous phone calls. Did not sleep last night, but is taking short naps during the day. _____M. Green, R.N.

1. The client is experiencing acute mania.
2. The client's bipolar mania is being effectively controlled with medication.
3. The client is experiencing extra-pyramidal side effects (EPS) from the medication.
4. The client needs prophylactic treatment for akathisia and tardive dyskinesia.

297. ANSWER: 2, 3, 4, 6.
Signs of oxcarbazepine toxicity include ataxia, sedation, diplopia, and dizziness. Excessive salivation and agitation are not associated with carbamazepine toxicity.

TEST-TAKING TIP: Focus on the options that suggest CNS depression.

Content Area: Mental Health; **Category of Health Alteration:** Pharmacological and Parenteral Therapies; **Integrated Processes:** Nursing Process Assessment; **Client Need:** Physiological Integrity/Pharmacological and Parenteral Therapies/ Adverse Effects/Contraindications/Interactions; **Cognitive Level:** Application; **Reference:** Fortinash, K., & Holoday Worret, P. (2008), pp. 561–562.

298. ANSWER: 3.
The nurse should conclude that the client is experiencing extra-pyramidal side effects of pacing, rocking, inability to sit still, lip smacking, and writhing movements of the fingers and toes. Acute mania is characterized by euphoria and elation, rapid thinking proceeding to racing and disoriented thinking, excessive psychomotor behavior with poor impulse control, such as with excessive spending or becoming sexually uninhibited. Easily distracted, going from one action to the next, making numerous phone calls, going without sleep but taking short naps during the day are associated with hypomania, suggesting the bipolar mania, and not acute mania, is not being effectively controlled. EPS of akathisia and tardive dyskinesia are not treated prophylactically.

TEST-TAKING TIP: Olanzapine is an atypical antipsychotic medication. Consider the side effect of EPS of this group of medications.

Content Area: Mental Health; **Category of Health Alteration:** Pharmacological and Parenteral Therapies; **Integrated Processes:** Communication and Documentation; **Client Need:** Physiological Integrity/Pharmacological and Parenteral Therapies/ Adverse Effects/Contraindications/Interactions; **Cognitive Level:** Analysis; **References:** Deglin, J., & Vallerand, A. (2009), pp. 1105–1107; Fortinash, K., & Holoday Worret, P. (2008), pp. 241–243; Varcarolis, E., & Halter, M. (2009), pp. 251–252.

299. After caring for a client for a number of days, a nurse on the mental health unit determines that lithium has been **ineffective** in treating a client's acute mania and that the client's behavior has been escalating. Place the symptoms in numerical order (1–6) observed by a nurse if the client's behavior is escalating from normal behavior to the most severe behavior of acute mania.

_____ 1. Becomes irritated easily

_____ 2. Speech is meaningful, coherent, and calm

_____ 3. Minimal sleep; writing lengthy letters and making many long-distance telephone calls

_____ 4. Demonstrates poor judgment and impulse control

_____ 5. Excessively cheerful and demonstrates boundless enthusiasm

_____ 6. Exaggerating achievements and believing he or she has great powers

300. A child diagnosed with attention deficit disorder is to receive a total of 20 mg of dextroamphetamine (Adderall) daily in two divided doses. The dextroamphetamine on hand is supplied in 5-mg tablets. How many tablet(s) should the nurse administer for the morning dose?

_____ tablet(s) (Record your answer as a whole number.)

299. ANSWER: 2, 5, 3, 1, 4, 6.

In normal behavior speech is meaningful, coherent, and calm. Then the client has increased sociability and euphoria (excessively cheerful and demonstrates boundless enthusiasm). When full blown, the client's activity level increases (minimal sleep, writing lengthy letters, and making many long-distance telephone calls). As the mania increases, the client becomes easily irritated and demonstrates poor judgment and impulse control. Exaggerating achievements and believing he or she has great powers indicate that the client has become psychotic and has delusions of grandeur.

TEST-TAKING TIP: First identify the normal behavior and then the progressively more severe behaviors.

Content Area: Mental Health; **Category of Health Alteration:** Pharmacological and Parenteral Therapies; **Integrated Processes:** Nursing Process Assessment; **Client Need:** Psychosocial Integrity/Mental Health Concepts; **Cognitive Level:** Analysis; **Reference:** Varcarolis, E., & Halter, M. (2009), pp. 250–253.

300. ANSWER: 2

First, determine the number of tablets for the total daily dose:

5 mg : 1 tablet :: 20 mg : X tablets.

$5X = 20$

$X = 4$ tablets.

The total daily dose of 20 mg would be 4 tablets. The order is two divided doses. Thus, divide the total number of 4 tablets by 2 to arrive at the number of tablets that should be administered.

TEST-TAKING TIP: First, determine the total dosage for the day, and then divide the total dose by 2 to determine the amount of each dose.

Content Area: Mental Health; **Category of Health Alteration:** Pharmacology and Parenteral Therapies; **Integrated Processes:** Nursing Process Planning; **Client Need:** Physiological Integrity/Pharmacological and Parenteral Therapies/Dosage Calculation; **Cognitive Level:** Analysis; **References:** Ball, J., & Bindler, R. (2008), p. 1116; Pickar, G., & Abernethy, A. (2008), p. 46.

Comprehensive Reference List

Aschenbrenner, D., & Venable, S. (2009). *Drug therapy in nursing* (3rd ed.). Philadelphia, PA: Lippincott Williams & Wilkins.

Ball, J., & Bindler, R. (2008). *Pediatric nursing: Caring for children* (4th ed.). Upper Saddle River, NJ: Prentice Hall/Pearson Education.

Berman, A., Snyder, S., Kozier, B., & Erb, G. (2008). *Kozier & Erb's fundamentals of nursing: Concepts, process, and practice* (8th ed.). Upper Saddle River, NJ: Pearson Education.

Berman, A., Snyder, S., & McKinney, D. (2011). *Nursing basics for clinical practice.* Upper Saddle River, NJ: Prentice Hall/Pearson Education.

Black, J., & Hawks, J. (2009). *Medical-surgical nursing: Clinical management for positive outcomes* (8th ed.). St. Louis, MO: Saunders/Elsevier.

Boyd, M. (2008). *Psychiatric nursing contemporary practice* (4th ed.). Philadelphia, PA: Lippincott Williams & Wilkins.

Chapman, L., & Durham, R. F. (2010). *Maternal-newborn nursing.* Philadelphia, PA: F.A. Davis.

Craven, R., & Hirnle, C. (2009). *Fundamentals of nursing: Human health and function* (6th ed.). Philadelphia: Lippincott Williams & Wilkins.

Davidson, M., London, M., & Ladewig, P. (2008). *Olds' maternal-newborn nursing & women's health across the lifespan* (8th ed.). Upper Saddle River, NJ: Prentice Hall Health.

Deglin, J., Vallerand, A., & Sanoski, C. (2011). *Davis's drug guide for nurses* (12th ed.). Philadelphia, PA: F.A. Davis.

Edelman, C., & Mandle, C. (2006). *Health promotion throughout the life span* (6th ed.). St. Louis, MO: Mosby/Elsevier.

Fortinash, K., & Holoday Worret, P. (2007). *Psychiatric nursing care plans* (5th ed.). St. Louis, MO: Mosby/Elsevier.

Fortinash, K., & Holoday Worret, P. (2008). *Psychiatric mental health nursing* (4th ed.). St. Louis, MO: Mosby/Elsevier.

Geiter, H. B. (2007). *E-Z ECG rhythm interpretation.* Philadelphia, PA: F.A. Davis.

Harkreader, H., Hogan, M., & Thobaben, M. (2007). *Fundamentals of nursing* (3rd ed.). St. Louis, MO: Saunders/Elsevier.

Ignatavicius, D., & Workman, M. (2010). *Medical-surgical nursing: Critical thinking for collaborative care* (6th ed.). St. Louis, MO. Elsevier/Saunders.

Kee, J. (2009). *Laboratory and diagnostic tests with nursing implications* (8th ed.). Upper Saddle River, NJ: Prentice Hall/Pearson Education.

Kyle, T. (2008). *Essentials of pediatric nursing.* Philadelphia, PA: Lippincott Williams & Wilkins.

Kneisl, C., & Trigoboff, E. (2009). *Contemporary psychiatric mental health nursing* (2nd ed.). Upper Saddle River, NJ: Prentice Hall/Pearson Education.

Lehne, R. (2007). *Pharmacology for nursing care* (6th ed.). St. Louis, MO: Saunders/Elsevier.

Lewis, S., Heitkemper, M., Dirksen, S., O'Brien, P., Bucher L., & Camera, I. (2011). *Medical-surgical nursing: Assessment and management of clinical problems* (8 th ed.). St. Louis, MO: Mosby/Elsevier.

Lutz, C., & Przytulski, K. (2011). *Nutrition & diet therapy: Evidence-based applications* (5th ed.). Philadelphia, PA: F.A. Davis.

Marquis, B. L., & Huston, C. J. (2009). *Leadership roles and management functions in nursing.* Philadelphia, PA: Lippincott Williams & Wilkins.

Mauk, K. (2010). *Gerontological nursing: Competencies for care* (2nd ed.). Sudbury, MA: Jones & Bartlett.

Myers, E. (2010). *RNotes* (3rd ed.). Philadelphia, PA: F.A. Davis.

Myers, E., & Hopkins, T. (2008). *MedSurg notes* (2nd ed.). Philadelphia, PA: F.A. Davis.

Osborn, S., Wraa, C., & Watson, A. (2010). *Medical-surgical nursing: Preparation for practice.* Upper Saddle River, NJ: Prentice Hall/Pearson Education.

Pedersen, D. (2008). *Psych notes* (2nd ed.). Philadelphia: F. A. Davis.

Perry, S., Hockenberry, M., Lowdermilk, D., & Wilson, D. (2010). *Maternal child nursing care* (4th ed.). St. Louis, MO: Mosby/Elsevier.

Phillips, L. (2010). *Manual of I.V. therapeutics* (5th ed.). Philadelphia, PA: F.A. Davis.

Pickar, G., & Abernethy, A. (2008). *Dosage calculations* (8th ed.). Clifton Park, NY: Thomson Delmar Learning.

Pillitteri, A. (2010). *Maternal & child health nursing: Care of the childbearing & childrearing family* (6th ed.). Philadelphia, PA: Lippincott Williams & Wilkins.

Potter, P., & Perry, A. (2009). *Fundamentals of nursing* (7th ed.). St. Louis, MO: Mosby/Elsevier.

Smeltzer, S., Bare, B., Hinkle, J., & Cheever, K. (2010). *Brunner & Suddarth's textbook of medical-surgical nursing* (12th ed.). Philadelphia, PA: Lippincott Williams & Wilkins.

Spratto, G., & Woods, A. (2010). *Delmar nurse's drug handbook: 2010 edition.* Clifton Park, NY: Delmar Cengage Learning.

Trigoboff, E. (2009). Substance related disorders. In C. Kneisl & E. Trigoboff, Eds., *Contemporary psychiatric mental health nursing* (2nd ed.). Upper Saddle River, NJ: Prentice Hall/Pearson Education.

Townsend, M. (2006). *Psychiatric mental health nursing: Concepts of care in evidence-based practice* (5th ed.). Philadelphia, PA: F.A. Davis.

Townsend, M. (2008). *Essentials of psychiatric mental health nursing* (4th ed.). Philadelphia, PA: F.A. Davis.

Townsend, M. (2009). *Psychiatric mental health nursing: Concepts of care in evidence-based practice* (6th ed.). Philadelphia, PA: F.A. Davis.

Townsend, M. (2011). *Essentials of psychiatric mental health nursing* (5th ed.). Philadelphia, PA: F.A. Davis.

Van Leeuwen, A., & Poelhuis-Leth, D. (2009). *Davis's comprehensive handbook of laboratory and diagnostic tests with nursing implications* (3rd ed.). Philadelphia, PA: F.A. Davis.

Varcarolis, E., & Halter, M. (2009). *Essentials of psychiatric mental health nursing.* St. Louis, MO: Saunders/Elsevier.

Ward, S., & Hisley, S. (2009). *Maternal-child nursing care.* Philadelphia, PA: F.A. Davis.

Whitehead, D., Weiss, S., & Tappen, R. (2010). *Essentials of nursing leadership and management* (5th ed.). Philadelphia, PA: F.A. Davis.

Wilkinson, J., & Treas, L. (2011a). *Fundamentals of nursing: Theory, concepts, & application* (2nd ed.). Philadelphia, PA: F.A. Davis.

Wilkinson, J., & Treas, L. (2011b). *Fundamentals of nursing: Thinking & doing* (2nd ed.). Philadelphia, PA: F.A. Davis.

Wilson, B., Shannon, M., Shields, K., & Stang, C. (2008). *Prentice hall nurse's drug guide 2008.* Upper Saddle River, NJ: Prentice Hall/Pearson Education.

Wilson, B., Shannon, M., & Shields, K. (2010). *Prentice hall nurse's drug guide 2010.* Upper Saddle River, NJ: Prentice Hall/Pearson Education.

Illustration Credits

Pages 113, 114, 145 from: De Castillo, S., & Werner-McCullough, M. (2007). *Student workbook to accompany calculating drug dosages* (2nd ed.). Philadelphia, PA: F.A. Davis.

Pages 35, 36, 91, 92, 109, 110, 111, 112, 117, 139 (lower right), 197, 211 (lower left) from: Dillon, P. (2007). *Nursing health assessment: A critical thinking, case studies approach* (2nd ed.). Philadelphia, PA: F.A. Davis.

Pages 7 (upper left), 139 (upper left, upper right, lower left), 211 (top left) from: Goldsmith, L.A., Lazarus, G.S., & Tharp, M.D. (1997). *Adult and pediatric dermatology*. Philadelphia, PA: F.A. Davis, with permission.

Pages 41, 42 from: Hockenberry, M., & Wilson, D. (2007). *Wong's nursing care of infants and children* (8th ed.). St. Louis, MO: Mosby/Elsevier, with permission.

Page 101 from: Holloway, B., Moredich, C., & Aduddell, K. (2006) *OB peds women's health notes: Nurse's clinical guide*. Philadelphia, PA: F.A. Davis.

Page 143 from: Jones, S. (2005). *ECG notes*. Philadelphia, PA: F.A. Davis.

Pages 15, 68, from Myers, E., & Hopkins, T. (2008). *Med-Surg Notes*. Philadelphia, PA: F.A. Davis.

Pages 7 (lower right), 8, 211 (top right) from: Reeves, J.R.T., & Maibach, H. (1991). *Clinical dermatology illustrated: A regional approach*. Philadelphia, PA: F.A. Davis.

Pages 31, 32, 49, 203, 204 from: Scanlon, V.C., & Sanders, T. (2007). *Essentials of anatomy and physiology* (5th ed). Philadelphia, PA: F.A. Davis.

Pages 301, 302 from: Townsend, M. (2006). *Psychiatric mental health nursing, concepts of care in evidence-based practice* (5th ed.). Philadelphia, PA: F.A Davis.

Pages 169 (bottom), 233, 234, 249 (top 4) from: Venes, D. [Ed.]. (2001). *Taber's cyclopedic medical dictionary* (19th ed.). Philadelphia, PA: F.A. Davis.

Pages 123, 227, 228, 249 (bottom), 255, 256, 257, 263 (upper left, lower left) from: Ward, S., & Hisley, S. (2009). *Maternal-child nursing care*. Philadelphia, PA: F.A. Davis.

Pages 3, 7 (upper right, lower left), 23, 27, 28, 81, 147, 157, 159, 160, 165, 166, 169 (top), 175, 176, 177, 178, 179, 189 (top row), 199, 211 (lower right), 239 from: Williams, L., & Hopper, P. (2007). *Understanding medical-surgical nursing*. Philadelphia: F.A. Davis.

Pages 73, 74, 185, 186, 189 (bottom row) from Wilkinson, J., & Van Leuven, K. (2007), *Fundamentals of nursing: Theory, concepts, & application* (Vol. 1). Philadelphia, PA: F.A. Davis.

Pages 17, 37, 39, 43, 44, 45, 51, 61, 62, 67, 77, 83, 84, 89, 193, 194, from: Wilkinson, J., & Van Leuven, K. (2007). *Fundamentals of nursing: Thinking & doing*. Philadelphia, PA: F.A. Davis.

Index

A

Family functioning assessment
  HIV infected-client in, 139-140
Feeding tubes
  medication administered through, 67-68
Fetal heart rate
  documentation of, 101-102
Fetal heart tones
  site of loudest, 91-92
Fetal movement counts
  teaching on, 97-98
Fetal scalp electrode placement
  indications for, 103-104
Fever
  in meningitis, 215-216
  pediatric, 55-56, 63-64
  postpartum, 109-110
Filgrastim
  dosage calculation of, 247-248
Financial exploitation
  in elder mistreatment, 137-138
Fine motor developmental milestones
  in children, 223-224
First aid
  to unresponsive accident victim, 87-88
Fluid loss
  in infant diarrhea, 51-52
Fluid therapy
  infusion calculation in pediatric, 271-272
  in pediatric gastroenteritis, 277-278
Fontanel palpation
  in infant head injury, 255-256
Fosphenytoin
  dosage calculation of, 275-276
Fundus
  postpartum location of, 111-112
Fungal infection
  foot, 31-32
  room assignments and, 17-18
Furosemide
  treatment of pediatric, 253-254
  dose calculation of, 57-58

G

Gastroduodenostomy
  teaching on, 159-160
Gastroenteritis
  in infant, 241-242
  treatment of pediatric, 277-278
Gastroesophageal reflux disease
  cimetidine in, 209-210
Gastrointestinal bleeding
  from peptic ulcer, 155-156
Gastrointestinal management
  in adults, 153-160
  in children, 239-242
Gastrostomy tube
  delegation and, 23-24
  medication administered through, 67-68
  procedural error in feeding through, 45-46
Genetic disorders
  hypertrophic cardiomyopathy as, 227-228
Genetic testing
  for sickle cell disease, 243-244
Gestational diabetes
  counseling in, 93-94
Glasgow coma scale
  in children, 257-258
Glaucoma
  client teaching on, 137-138
Glove and gown removal
  after contact isolation procedures, 89-90
Graves' disease
  pharmacotherapy for, 211-212, 237-238
Growth and development
  in children, 223-226

H

Hallucinations
  therapeutic responses to, 291-292
Haloperidol
  dosage calculation of, 311-312
  side effects of, 295-296